BREAKING
THE CODE

A LAYPERSON'S GUIDE TO UNLOCKING THE SECRET WORLD OF MEDICAL TERMINOLOGY

by Dr. Richard Schulze

NATURAL HEALING
PUBLICATIONS

Published by Natural Healing Publications
P.O. Box 3628, Santa Monica. California 90408
1-877-TEACH-ME (832-2463)

Breaking The Code: A Layperson's Guide To Unlocking
The Secret World Of Medical Terminology

ISBN: 0-9671568-3-4

FIRST EDITION

WARNING

A WARNING from our Lawyers:

This book is published under the First Amendment of the United States Constitution, which grants the right to discuss openly and freely all matters of public concern and to express viewpoints no matter how controversial or unaccepted they may be. However, Medical groups and Pharmaceutical companies have finally infiltrated and violated our sacred Constitution. Therefore we are forced to give you the following WARNINGS:

If you are ill or have been diagnosed with any disease, please consult a medical doctor before attempting any natural healing program.

Many foods, herbs or other natural substances can occasionally have dangerous allergic reactions or side effects in some people. People have even died from allergic reactions to peanuts and strawberries.

Any one of the programs in this book could be potentially dangerous, even lethal, especially if you are seriously ill.

Therefore, any natural method you learn about in this book may cause harm, instead of the benefit you seek. ASK YOUR DOCTOR FIRST, but remember that the vast majority of doctors have no education in natural healing methods and herbal medicine. They will probably discourage you from trying any of the programs.

It usually starts with a little pain that you have ignored for a few years, but you are too busy to deal with it right now, you don't have the time, it will probably go away, but it doesn't . . .

10:00 a.m. So you made an appointment to have your medical doctor just take a look at it. It's probably nothing. But when the doctor takes a look you can see the concerned and worried look on their face. Your doctor says, "how long have you been experiencing this pain?", or "how long have you noticed this lump?" or "how long have you noticed this tingling?", or "dizziness", or "ringing in the ears", or "change in your bowel, or urination", or this "little cough". Then the doctor asks you to go in for numerous further tests, blood tests, a CT scan or an MRI, even a surgical biopsy, **THIS AFTERNOON.**

2:00 p.m. You arrive at the diagnostic lab. You try to get your insurance agent on your cell phone but they are not in. You go into a small room where you are told to strip off all your clothes and get on a table to have radioactive dye injected into your body, get strapped down and put inside a whirling machine (and you thought the CT scan was just a Polaroid.) Or you have to be sedated and have cameras and surgical tools put up your anus into your colon. The technician says that the procedure will be a *little* uncomfortable, but a root canal is looking like a walk in the park right now. You are terrified and in pain.

4:00 p.m. The results are positive, which means you're in trouble and the doctor says that you need immediate surgery and there is no time to waste. You could die if you wait even a day. It may be too late already. The surgery isn't a sure thing; it could even kill you, but you need to get on the operating table **RIGHT NOW!** The doctor leaves for a minute.

4:02 p.m. What did they say I had? What was the name of that disease? I've never even heard of that organ. Is all of this really necessary? Should I get a second opinion? Maybe my doctor just needs money for a balloon payment on his mortgage. How much does my insurance cover? Is my will up to date? Where did I put it? Your doctor comes into the room and tells you that arrangements have been made and asks you to go to the hospital and admit yourself, **NOW.**

Every day I hear this same story. People in pain with diseases have anxiety, uncertainty, confusion, and are forced to make rushed, life and death decisions that might cost them their life savings or put them in debt forever, that might even kill them, and they don't even know what the test results meant and literally have no idea what the doctor was talking about.

Breaking the Code is all about giving the patient MORE TIME.

No decision has to be made in five minutes or even that day. Take the time to look up the words that you do not understand. Take the time to get familiar with the organs and systems in question, how they work and what they do. Take the time to decipher your tests results and possibly even get a second opinion but better yet, **consider an _alternative/natural_ opinion.** There are always options.

In my clinic I saw that there was rarely any real rush, that you had days, even weeks and months. After all, how long did you ignore your symptoms and how long did it take for your body to develop this disease? How long have you had it? Remember yesterday before the doctor terrified and tortured you? You weren't so bad off were you?

What I suggested to all of my patients was take a few weeks off, study what is supposedly wrong with you and learn more about those organs and systems that are in need, so you can make a more informed decision. And during those few weeks or a month that you are learning more about yourself, **get on an aggressive Natural Healing program.** Why not take an aggressive _natural_ approach before taking an aggressive and dangerous _surgical_ or _chemical_ approach? It just makes good common sense to see if a tune up fixes your car before you consider dissecting and rebuilding your entire engine.

In my clinic, on my aggressive healthy lifestyle changes, my patients would be feeling better in just a few days. If I could get my patients to give me a month, they were noticeably better, and if I could get them to give me three months, well they saved themselves a lot of pain, torture and money.

Breaking the Code is all about being informed so you can make better decisions.
What you will discover is that all the 20 dollar words aren't so scary once you figure out that **acute hyperhidrosis** just means you sweat a lot.

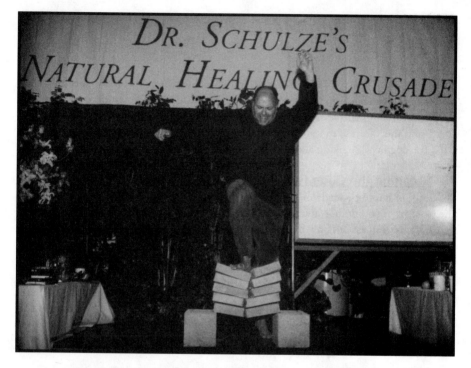

COMMON SENSE HEALING, *NATURALLY*
by Dr. Richard Schulze

POISON A PERSON WELL?

My clinic spanned three decades and I saw thousands and thousands of patients during that time. Most people do not choose Natural Healing and Herbal Medicine first.

My patients would walk into my clinic stunned, shocked and confused. They had supposedly done everything right, spent tens, even hundreds of thousands of dollars on the smartest doctors, the most educated specialists, the best hospitals with the latest equipment and the most advanced technology and the most potent modern smart-bomb chemical medicine. My patients even had the finest surgeons snip, clip and burn away all the bad parts. But their diseases returned. I would help them understand that <u>trying to poison, cut and burn yourself back to health might give temporary relief, but never creates true healing and health.</u> When the underlying cause of disease is not dealt with, the disease eventually returns. This is why with medical treatment, cancer always comes back, cleared coronary arteries get blocked again and all disease eventually returns. I would often ask a patient who underwent major medical treatment for disease, "What did <u>YOU</u> do to change your life so that you would not create this disease in your body again?" And most patients would look at me with a dumb stare like what the heck is he talking about?

My patients had handed over all of the responsibility for their health to their medical doctors. After all, the medical doctors assured them that they could fix everything, like new again. That they would be fine and that after their treatment they could *go out and enjoy themselves*, and do all the things that they used to do. What the medical doctors didn't bother to mention is that the *things they used to do* are what caused their diseases in the first place and that if they continued to live their lives that way, their diseases will not only return, but will most likely kill them the second time around.

TRUST ME, I'M A DOCTOR.

What is worse, is that my patients trusted and believed in their medical doctors so much they didn't ever bother to really learn or understand what was wrong with them in the first place. I would ask my patients, "What was the most important thing in your life?" Often they would say their family, or their career, or their house, but what could be more important than your health which lets you enjoy EVERYTHING? Without your health, without your physical body, you are physically DEAD and you can't enjoy ANYTHING. Most of my patients knew much more about their stock portfolios, car engines, fashion trends, hobbies, exotic cuisine, sports statistics, feng shui, specialized coffee drinks and sushi than they knew about their own body and how to care for it. This is just plain stupid and ignorant. Understanding how our body works and then learning how to care for it best is critical knowledge that we should have learned in grade school, long before reading, writing and arithmetic. Well we didn't.

WHAT THE HECK HAPPENED TO ME?

Now my patients were standing, trembling at my clinic door. They were broke, in pain, tortured and their damn disease came back and they were sick again. What's worse is that they didn't even really know what hit them. They had piles of papers, medical bills, medical files, lab tests, biopsy reports, surgical reports and many even had pictures, ultrasounds, CT scans, MRI's, even x-rays. But they didn't have the faintest idea what all of this medical trash meant. They were dazed and confused.

Besides helping them start a new life and heal themselves, often my job at first was to try to make some sense of this medical mayhem and explain in common sense plain English what the medical doctors were talking about. That's assuming the medical doctors knew what they were doing- which often they did not.

So now I not only had to help them heal themselves, but also try to educate them in what went wrong in the first place. Fixing the problem is of vital importance, but fixing the cause so it won't happen again runs a close second. The latter is the fundamental difference between Medical Healing and Natural Healing.

ABOUT THIS BOOK, BREAKING THE CODE

Every other month I write a GET WELL Newsletter. In each of these newsletters I cover a different subject, usually a system of the human body, the anatomy and physiology of this system, what common ways this system gets sick, its diseases, and how to heal this system naturally. I get hundreds of letters from people thanking me for teaching them about the organs and systems in a way that they can understand and also empowering them to heal themselves. Once I break down the twenty dollar words, all of this medical mumbo-jumbo is not that hard to understand.

One of the best ways to help my patients understand all of their medical reports was to help them understand the language of medicine. This book is a compilation of what I used in my clinic that best helped my patients decipher the words that the medical doctors use and understand the organs and systems of the body.

PREFIXES, ROOTS AND SUFFIXES

In this chapter are the parts of words that often make up the bigger medical words, the beginnings, the middles and the endings. For instance Nephritis is the combination of <u>Nephr</u> (from the Greek Nephros) meaning Kidney and <u>itis</u> (another from the Greek) meaning inflammation. Hence Nephritis means Kidney Inflammation. So if you have said in the past, referring to medical terminology, "it's all Greek to me" you were literally correct.

ANATOMY, PHYSIOLOGY AND THE DESCRIPTIONS OF SYSTEMS

In this chapter I describe in simple terms, the major systems of the body, the important organs that are generally included in these systems, how these organs work and what they do. Along with each system I include a glossary of words that are often used by doctors to describe these particular organs, systems and the diseases thereof.

A FEW MORE BOOKS THAT CAN HELP

A good medical dictionary can help you a lot. One of the better ones is Taber's Cyclopedic Medical Dictionary. This is a standard on almost every medical doctor's desk so they can understand what the heck the other medical doctors are talking about.

Also a copy of the Physicians Desk Reference is very helpful. This is the grand book of drugs. This book helps you look up every pharmaceutical drug by brand name, chemical name, manufacturer's name and even by picture. What's much better is its over THREE THOUSAND PAGES of the most horrifying information about all the things that can go wrong if you dare swallow this chemical poison, and best yet, it is written by the drug manufacturers themselves. In the clinic I would simply make a copy of the two or three pages describing each drug that my patients were taking. I never needed to say any more. The horrors of chemical medicine are well documented under cautions, precautions, adverse reactions, and contraindications.

Often I would discover that the medications my patients were prescribed and taking were contraindicated for them because of some preexisting disease or not to be mixed with the other medications that they were on. I would also often find that their dosage suggested was much higher than what the manufacturer considered safe.

My patients had been prescribed drugs for their diseases, like <u>Beta Cell Blockers</u> (which anesthetize the beta cell nerve receptors on the heart muscle), for their heart disease like cardiac arrhythmia (irregular heart beat) only to discover that they first were taking medication for a sinus infection prescribed by a different doctor that contains chemicals that are <u>Beta Cell Stimulants</u>. In other words the side effects of their first drug caused their second, and more deadly *disease*, and their stupid medical doctor who didn't take the time to do a complete history during the two minute office visit never asked what drugs they were currently taking and prescribed them a second, more powerful and dangerous drug that could literally kill them, to combat not a disease, but the side effects of the previous drug they were prescribed.

Every day in my clinic I would see patients that were well, but made sick by their medication, and when I took them off their chemical drugs, they miraculously got well.

FOCUS ON CREATING HEALTH

<u>Always remember, you do not have to know any of this to heal yourself of any disease.</u> This information is supplied for those that are interested in deciphering medical reports, tests, articles, whatever.

In reality, diagnosis is poor at best. Often medical statistics show that top medical specialists and leading diagnostic hospitals are only correct in their diagnoses, 15% of the time. Where does that put your average medical doctor? 10% correct. You could get better results with a monkey spinning a bottle or flipping a coin. Also medical, biopsy, surgical and pathology reports are often wrong. Every week in my clinic I would find that in a patient's medical report the doctor described the ultrasound results as a tumor being three inches in diameter, the size of an orange. But in the surgical report it was hard to discern whether a tumor existed in the body at all or that it was just some unknown benign tissues. By the time the pathology report was written, there was nothing but a little tissue to report. What happened to this gigantic tumor? Did the surgeon lose it on the way to pathology? Did it ever exist? Will you ever know? I have had many surgeons confide in me that once they opened up the patient, what they thought was there from the tests and ultrasounds was not there at all. But they don't tell this to the patient.

I want you to understand that more often than not, in my clinic I found that the medical doctor's diagnosis was wrong, if not absurd. I also discovered that even if the diagnosis was correct, the prognosis of what will happen to you is based on your continuing to be the physically, emotionally and spiritually sick and degenerate average American.

With this in mind, don't take your diagnosis, your medical tests and reports, and your disease for that matter, too seriously. Put your focus, time and energy into creating a healthy lifestyle rather than understanding your medical reports. Experience how it feels to be really healthy and alive instead of studying your disease, and before you know it, you will be well.

Dr. Richard Schulze

TABLE OF CONTENTS

TABLE OF CONTENTS

CHAPTER 1

GLOSSARY OF GENERAL MEDICAL TERMS

PREFIXES – *a group of letters put before a word, changing or modifying its meaning (ex: cardiac arrythmia – cardiac=heart,* **a=without**, *rythmia=rhythm or* **heart** <u>**without**</u> **rhythm**)

A-, An-	without. Anosmia – no sense of smell
Auto-	self
Bi –	two, double or twice
Dys-	bad, abnormal, difficult
Endo-	usually refers to the inside lining of an organ. Endoscopy
Exo-	outside of; without
Hemi-	half or a portion of. Hemiplegia – paralysis of one half of the body
Hyper-	over, too much. Hyperthyroidism, hyperpyrexia
Hypo-	under, too little. Hypothyroidism
Inter-	between
Intra-	inside
Macro-	large or long
Micro-	small
Nul –	none
Oligo –	few, small
Poly –	many, much, excess. Polydipsia – excessive thirst (as in diabetes). Polymyositis – inflammation of many muscles

ROOTS – *the main body of a word. The practice of medicine is ancient so the terminology used is from some very old and rarely used languages like Latin, Old English, and archaic dialects of Greek, French and even Spanish. So all we are going to do is decipher some foreign languages...*

Amnio	pertaining to the innermost fetal membrane in the womb that holds the fetus suspended in fluid
Arthr	pertaining to the joints. Arthrosis, arthritis.
Benign	not recurrent or progressive; not malignant
Calculus	stone. biliary, renal calculus. Acalculus cholecystitis
Cardio	pertaining to the heart
Centesis	puncture of an organ to relieve pressure. Thoracentesis, pleuracentesis, amniocentesis,
cephal	brain. Encephalitis
cervical	pertaining to the neck or to the cervix
chole	bile. Cholesterol – bile solid (steros=solid), cholestasis, hypercholesterolemia
chondro	cartilage
colic	spasm in any hollow or tubular soft organ accompanied by pain
colon	the large intestine. Colonoscopy
costo	pertaining to the rib
cryo	cold, freezing. Cryosurgery, cryotherapy – procedures involving freezing of tissues
cyto	cell
cyst	closed sac or pouch that contains fluid, fluid like or solid material; cystitis – inflammation of a cyst; cholecystitis – inflammation of a cyst containing bile
edema	swelling

epithelio	pertaining to outer layer of the skin (the epidermis) or the surface layer of mucous membranes
esophageal	referring to the esophagus
fibro	structural tissue that connect organs to each others, usually containing, collagen, elastin, proteins.fibromyalgia
flexure	bend. Hepatic flexure
gastro	pertaining to the stomach
hemo	blood
hepatic	referring to the liver
infarction	refers to an area of tissue that dies due to a blockage of the blood supply to that area. Ex: myocardial infarction – heart attack
leuko	pertaining to the white blood cells
lipo	fat. Lipoma – tumor made of fat cells
lith	stone. Cholelithiasis – condition of having stones in the gallbladder
lucent	transparent
lymph	colorless, alkaline fluid found in the lymphatic vessels of the body consisting mainly of proteins, salts, fats, fluid, white blood cells and other organic substances; also, pertaining to white blood cells
lyse	to kill
malignant	tending or threatening to produce death; harmful. Used to refer to cancerous growths
media	middle. Otitis media – infection of the middle ear
meno	pertaining to menstruation
meninges	linings of the spinal cord and brain
metro	uterus

mycosis	fungal infection or condition. Onychomycosis – fungal infection of the nail
myelo	spinal cord or bone marrow
myo	muscle
nephr	kidney. Pyelonephritis – infection of the kidney(s)
neuro	pertaining to neurons, the nerves, the nervous system
noct	pertaining to nighttime
nosocomial	pertaining to or occurring in a hospital
oligo	little, scant, not much
onycho	of the fingernail or toenail
oophor	(Greek oophoros – bearing eggs) ovary
orch	testicle. Orchitis – inflammation/infection of the testicle
osteo	bone. Osteoporosis – reduction in bone density resulting in fractures, pain, etc. Osteomyelitis - infection of the bone and the bone marrow. Osteodystrophy – defective bone development
oto	ear. Otitis media – middle ear infection
parity	the condition of having carried a pregnancy to the point of a fetal weight of 500 grams or 20 weeks gestation
pepsia	to digest. Dyspepsia – difficult digestion
phage	to swallow. Phagocyte – cell that swallows. Dysphagia – difficulty swallowing
phasia	speech. Dysphasia – difficult speech. Aphasia – without speech
phleb	vein. Phlebitis – inflammation/infection of the vein
plegia	paralysis

pleur	refers to the membrane that lines both lungs. Pleuritis – inflammation of the lung lining
pnea	air, breathing. Apnea – lack of breathing. Dyspnea – difficulty breathing
pneumo	gas, air, respiration, lung. Pneumothorax – abnormal presence of air in the thorax; also called collapsed lung
polyp	a tumor with a pedicle, commonly found in the nose, uterus, colon and rectum
pyo	pus. Pyuria – pus in the urine
pyrexia	fever
renal	pertaining to the kidney
rhino	nose. Rhinitis, rhinoplasty
salpinx	fallopian tube. Pyosalpinx – infection causing pus in the Fallopian tubes.
sarco	flesh. Sarcoid – resembling flesh. Sarcoidosis – condition of having fleshy tumors
sclerosis	hardening usually due to excessive growth of tissue. Arteriosclerosis – hardening of the arteries; Multiple sclerosis
septic	pertaining to pathogenic organisms or their toxins
splen	pertaining to the spleen. Splenectomy – surgical removal of the spleen
stasis	no movement; stagnant. Cholestasis – stagnant bile in the liver/gall bladder
stenosis	abnormal narrowing of a passageway in the body
thorac	thorax; that part of the body between the base of the neck and the diaphragm; thoracotomy, thoracentesis, etc.
trophy	from trophe – nourishment; growth of an organ. Hypertrophy – increase in size of organ due to growth not a tumor; atrophy – a wasting away or decrease in size of an organ usually due to disuse

SUFFIXES – *a group of letters put after a word, changing or modifying its meaning. (ex: hepatitis – hepatic=liver,* **itis=inflammation,** *or liver* **inflammation**)

-atic	stops growth. Bacteriostatic – stops growth of bacteria
-cide	killing. Bactericide – kills bacteria; fungicide, pesticide, etc.
-ectomy	surgical removal. Appendectomy, cholecystectomy, hysterectomy, prostatectomy, etc.
-emia	in or of the blood. Septicemia – pathogenic microorganisms in the blood, Anemia – without blood
-genic	arising from; caused by. Somatogenic, psychogenic
-iasis	condition. Nephrolithiasis – condition of having stones in the kidney(s)
-itis	inflammation or infection
-oma	tumor. Lipoma – fat cell tumor. Adenoma – tumor of a gland cell. Lymphoma, carcinoma, sarcoma
-oscopy	skopein (to examine), scope used to examine the inside of the body. Sigmoidoscopy, colonoscopy, colposcopy, etc.
-osis	condition, usually abnormal
-ostomy	surgical formed artificial opening
-otomy	surgical incision
-pathy	disease. Osteopathy – disease of the bones
-penia	deficiency; lack of. Leukopenia – not enough white blood cells
-plasty	plastic surgery. Rhinoplasty – plastic surgery of the nose
-rrhagia	hemorrhage; bleeding. Menorrhagia – excessive menstrual flow
-rrhea	to flow. Menorrhea – menstrual flow. Diarrhea
-taxis	attracting or repelling movement
-uria	pertaining to the urine; see urinary system terms

CHAPTER 2

THE DIGESTIVE, ASSIMILATION AND ELIMINATION SYSTEM

EXPLANATION OF SYSTEM

*Thousands of patients walked into my clinic with **stomach** aches, but when I would ask them where their **stomach** hurt, they would almost always point to their **colon** instead, **about 12 inches below their stomach!** We walk around in our body for a hundred years but have little or no idea where our particular organs are. Well not anymore. I will show you where your digestive system and colon are and put an end to the mystery.*

Your colon is the last stage of your digestive tract and has many jobs. Having a basic understanding of your colon's functions can keep you healthy and prevent disease.

THE 30 FOOT LONG JOURNEY

I will take the liberty here of actually describing the entire digestive and elimination tract. The main reason for this is I don't know the next time I will get close to this subject and it may be helpful to many of you to understand the upper gastro-intestinal anatomy and physiology. And as always, if this section is more than you can comprehend, drop it. There will be no test, and you can heal yourself of anything without knowing the following information. Saying that . . .

The digestive and elimination tract is one long tube from your mouth to your anus, just shy of thirty feet long. There is only one way in and one way out. This tube is often referred to as the **alimentary canal** or tract which includes the **mouth, esophagus, stomach, duodenum, small intestine, large intestine, rectum** and **anus**.

When you chew, saliva is produced in your mouth from the salivary glands and mixes with food. This is often referred to as the first stage of digestion because saliva enzymes initiate the digestion of starches. Saliva also lubricates the food for its initial travel down the esophagus. The **ESOPHAGUS**, about nine inches long, takes swallowed food down to your stomach. Where the esophagus meets the stomach there is an **esophageal sphincter muscle** which relaxes to let food enter the **stomach** and then contracts to prevent the backup of stomach contents.

The **STOMACH.** It is a muscular sac with a mucosa lining. This lining secretes gastric juices like hydrochloric acid and pepsin, that help to further digest your food. These juices start the digestion of proteins. Just the sight and smell of food triggers the excretion of gastric juices. Bad habits, like chewing gum continually, stimulate and fool the stomach into thinking food is on the way and can lead to digestive and stomach trouble. Also animal foods, especially beef and pork, are almost impossible to digest and require the constant secretion of acid which can lead to stomach and duodenal ulcers, burnt tissue and eventually holes in your stomach and intestinal lining. *(OK, I know I strayed to natural healing and not anatomy and physiology.)*

At the end of the stomach is the **pyloric valve**, which keeps the stomach's contents in the stomach until they are sufficiently processed and digested to move on. This valve and the emptying of the stomach's contents are triggered by hormones, nerves and other factors.

The **SMALL INTESTINE.** As food is released from the stomach through the pyloric valve it enters the **duodenum** which is technically considered the first part of the small intestine. The duodenum is almost a foot long. When partially digested food, sometimes referred to as **chyme,** enters the duodenum it triggers the release of hormones. These **digestive hormones** are released from the walls of the duodenum and stimulate the **liver** and **gallbladder** to release **bile** which enters the duodenum through the **common bile duct.** These hormones also stimulate the **pancreas** to release **pancreatic juices** into the duodenum through the same common bile duct, sometimes referred to as the pancreatic duct. <u>These liver and pancreatic juices continue the process from the stomach of breaking down carbohydrates and proteins but now these juices also start to break down fats.</u> The walls of the duodenum secrete digestive juices too.

The second part of the small intestine is called the **jejunum** which is about nine feet long and the third and last part of the small intestine is called the **ileum** which is thirteen feet long and terminates at the **illeocecal valve** at the beginning of the colon or large intestine. The wall of the entire small intestine (all three parts) is folded and looks like accordion pleats. These folds have even smaller folds on their surface called **villi,** which are small projections about 3/8 of an inch long. There are even **micro-villi** that are smaller. Obviously all of these folds increase the surface area of the small intestine. Since this is where the majority of food absorption takes place, the more surface area to absorb, the better. Each **villus** (the singular of villi) contains a capillary network which introduces the digested food nutrients into your bloodstream. The **portal vein** transports this digested food first to your liver and then if deemed acceptable, onward into your entire circulatory system to feed every cell in your body.

At the end of the small intestine is the **illeocecal valve** which allows food to pass into the large intestine,

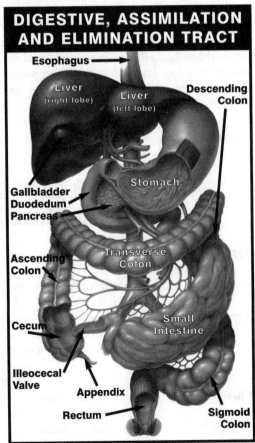

DIGESTIVE, ASSIMILATION AND ELIMINATION TRACT

Esophagus

Liver (right lobe)

Liver (left lobe)

Descending Colon

Gallbladder
Duodedum
Pancreas

Stomach

Ascending Colon

Transverse Colon

Cecum

Small Intestine

Illeocecal Valve

Appendix

Rectum

Sigmoid Colon

colon or bowel, whichever you want to call it. The **LARGE INTESTINE** is about five feet long and seven inches in circumference. It has no villi but still can absorb water, vitamins and minerals from the intestinal contents. This process dries the intestinal contents and turns them into waste, **fecal matter**, for release or defecation.

The first part of the large intestine is called the **cecum**. The **vermiform appendix**, about three to four inches long, is right below the illeocecal valve. It is an immune system aggregation similar to the tonsils, adenoids and the Peyer's patches in the small intestine. Here is the perfect placement to detect any pathogen or microorganism that may be harmful to you as the digested food enters the final stage of digestion, ready for elimination. This is also the biggest anti-gravity and uphill trek for the food. The vermiform appendix also excretes fluids that lubricate the food and stimulate peristalsis, the muscular contractions of the colon that move the food and eventually fecal matter along. The parts of the large intestine are referred to in order, **cecum**, **ascending colon**, **hepatic flexure** (the first turn near the liver), **transverse colon**, **spleenic flexure** (downward bend near the spleen), **descending colon**, **sigmoid colon**, **rectum** and **anus**. Parasites are often found in the cecum and in the appendix. It is their favorite breeding ground and hiding place. Constipation, on the other hand, is most often found in the descending and sigmoid colon. The rectum is about five inches long and is considered the end of the colon. The anus is the sphincter muscle at the end of the rectum that opens to release the undigested and unassimilated food residue called feces, fecal matter, stool or excrement. I don't know who was the first person to take a good look at and examine feces, *probably a guy like me*, but in any case, examination of the stool is a diagnostic art in itself. Color, form, consistency, odor, and the presence of blood, mucous, parasites can all tell a story about a patient's health and have been used by doctors for centuries to diagnose disease. Still today, medical doctors use a stool sample to detect colon cancer and many other diseases.

GLOSSARY OF DIGESTIVE SYSTEM TERMINOLOGY

Appendectomy   surgical removal of the appendix performed in cases of appendicitis

Appendicitis   inflammation/infection of the appendix

Appendix   a long, narrow, hollow worm-shaped structure that projects from the end of the first part of the large intestine, the cecum, and lined with the same mucous membrane as the cecum; also called the vermiform appendix

Cholesterol   a sterol widely distributed in animal tissues and occurring in egg yolks, animal fats and oils, the nerve tissue of the brain and spinal cord, the liver, the kidneys, and the adrenal glands. It also can be made in the liver, and is normally present in the bile. The body uses cholesterol to make sex hormones (progesterone, testosterone, estrogen, etc.) Cholesterol is only found in the cell membranes of animal tissues and not in plants. It is the primary component of gallstones.

Colectomy   surgical removal of the colon

Colostomy   a surgical procedure whereby a portion of the colon is opened and connected to the outside surface of the body. A bag is glued to the outside opening of the body to catch the fecal contents which spill out the opening. A temporary or permanent surgery performed due to particular bowel diseases

Colon cancer   malignant tumor of the large intestine

Corticosteroids   type of medicinal steroid used to suppress the immune system. They are used to treat many diseases in which the immune system is considered overactive, like Crohn's disease and ulcerative colitis.

Crohn's Disease   inflammatory bowel disease marked by chronic inflammation, scarring, severe diarrhea, infection, and sometimes bleeding of the bowel

Diverticulosis   abnormal condition of the intestines marked by the presence of multiple diverticuli, or bowel pockets caused by a weakening of the muscular walls of the colon which is caused by years of constipation. The bowel pockets fill with old stagnant fecal material and can become inflamed and infected.

Diverticulitis   inflammation/infection of the diverticula in a person who has diverticulosis. The symptoms are diarrhea and bleeding of the intestines.

Duodenal ulcer   commonly called a stomach ulcer. A breakdown of the lining of the first part of the small intestine just past the stomach. Symptoms are indigestion, weakness, and pain in the stomach area. In severe cases, the ulcer can bleed.

Duodenum   first part of the small intestine that begins just after the stomach

Dyspepsia   (dys – painful, peptein – to digest) – difficult or painful digestion often described as indigestion, gaseousness, fullness or pain that is gnawing or burning felt in the upper abdomen or chest

Esophagus	muscular tube that carries swallowed foods and liquids from the pharynx to the stomach. At the junction with the stomach is the lower esophageal or cardiac sphincter, which relaxes to permit passage of food, then contracts to prevent backup of the contents of the stomach.
GERD	(pronounced gurd) short for gastroesophageal reflux disease; the abnormal backward flow of the contents of the stomach into the esophagus causing symptoms of heartburn, fullness, nausea and vomiting
Hemicolectomy	removal of half or less of the colon
Hemorrhoids	mass of dilated veins in the anorectal area caused by long term straining on the toilet and constipation. Internal hemorrhoids are usually painless and bleed. External ones are painful, itch, and do not bleed.
Hemotochezia	bright red blood in the stool. Usually indicates bleeding in the lower intestinal tract (large intestine, rectum)
Ileum	third or last part of the small intestine right before the beginning of the colon
Irritable Bowel Syndrome	probably a catchall term for digestive problems that are not easily diagnosed. It is usually characterized by abdominal pain and by alternating periods of constipation and diarrhea.
Jejunum	second part of the small intestine right after the duodenum and before the ileum
Melena	black, tarry looking feces caused by bleeding in the intestines. The red color of blood is changed to black during its passage through the intestines. It usually indicates bleeding in the upper intestinal tract (esophagus, stomach, small intestines)
Pancreatitis	inflammation of the pancreas
Pancreatic cancer	malignant tumor of the pancreas
Peyer's Patches	collection of lymph nodules found mainly in the ileum near its junction with the colon.

Spastic Colon	most frequently seen bowel disease marked by pain, abdominal cramping, and constipation alternating with diarrhea
Splenectomy	surgical removal of the spleen usually in the case of trauma or certain blood disorders
Triple therapy	combination of three medications used to treat ulcers
Ulcerative Colitis	inflammatory bowel disease in which the lining of the colon breaks down and is eliminated in the form of bloody diarrhea. The disease goes through periods of remission and exacerbation.

SPECIFIC HERBAL FORMULAE FOR THE DIGESTIVE SYSTEM

DR. SCHULZE'S INTESTINAL FORMULA #1

BOTANICAL INGREDIENTS *Curacao and Cape Aloe leaf, Aloe barbadensis and Aloe capensis or ferox,* **Senna leaves and pods,** *Cassia officinalis,* **Cascara Sagrada aged bark,** *Rhamnus purshiana,* **Barberry root bark,** *Berberis vulgaris,* **Ginger rhizome,** *Zingiber officinalis,* **Garlic bulb,** *Allium sativum,* **and Habanero peppers,** *Capsicum species.*

METABOLIC ACTION AND BOTANICAL CHEMISTRY A sluggish, constipated, swollen bowel, retaining pounds of old fecal matter can either compress a nearby area causing disease, or emit infection and toxins which can affect and infect any area of the body. This explains why about 80% of my patients that came into my clinic healed their heart problems, blood pressure problems, breathing problems, blood sugar problems, hormone imbalance problems, fertility problems, liver problems, cholesterol problems, immune problems, urinary problems, adrenal and lack of energy problems, prostate problems, digestive problems, lower back problems, leg circulation and nerve problems, the list is almost endless.

This stimulating tonic is cleansing, healing and strengthening to the entire gastro-intestinal system. It stimulates your peristaltic action (the muscular movement of the colon) and over time strengthens the muscles of the large intestine. It halts putrefaction and disinfects, soothes and heals the mucous membrane lining of your entire digestive tract. This herbal tonic improves digestion, relieves gas and cramps, increases the flow of bile which in turn cleans the gallbladder, bile ducts and liver, destroys Candida albicans overgrowth and promotes a healthy intestinal flora. It also destroys and expels intestinal parasites, increases gastro-intestinal circulation and is anti-bacterial, anti-viral and anti-fungal.

Aloe, Senna and Cascara Sagrada all contain colon stimulating phytochemicals called anthraquinones. The particular one common to all three of these herbs is called emodin, often referred to as aloe-emodin and sometimes as 1,8-dihydroxy-anthracene or numerous other similar names. Herbs that contain these chemicals, when ingested, increase peristaltic waves; the muscular contractions or propulsive contractions of the colon muscle. This results in fecal matter being accelerated through the colon. This action over time, with proper diet and positive lifestyle can strengthen the colon muscle to where these herbs are no longer needed to achieve normal bowel movements. **Barberry** contains bitter alkaloids, one of which is berberine. This phytochemical stimulates the liver, the gallbladder and the production of bile, which makes it a laxative to the hepatic system. **Garlic** is anti-bacterial, anti-viral and anti-fungal. Often when constipation has occurred, infection is present. Garlic's numerous sulfur compounds destroy harmful pathogens on contact and also help increase intestinal microflora. Finally **Capsicum and Ginger** are both powerful stimulants to the colon. Cayenne will also correct intestinal bleeding and Ginger increases *downward* peristalsis, stimulating every aspect of your digestion and elimination.

DOSAGE

DOSAGE FOR PATIENT TYPE A: *The sluggish bowel type.* This is about 98% of Americans, the ones who need help getting their bowels working more frequently. Start with only 1 capsule of this formula during or just after dinner. This formula works best when taken with food. The next morning you should notice an increase in your bowel action and in the amount of fecal matter that you eliminate. The consistency should also be softer. If you do not notice any difference in your bowel behavior by the next day, or if the difference was not dramatic, then that evening increase your dosage to 2 capsules. You can continue to increase your dosage every evening by one capsule until you notice a dramatic difference in the way your bowel works. There is no limit. Most people need only 2-3 capsules, but a few have needed over 30 capsules. It has taken most of us years to create a sluggish bowel, so let's be patient for a few days and increase by only 1 capsule each day. This formula can be taken for a week, a month or the rest of your life. Continue to use this formula until you are having one bowel movement each day for every meal you eat. Between two and four bowel movements a day is normal.

DOSAGE FOR PATIENT TYPE B: *The active, overactive or irritated bowel type.* This only applied to about 2% of my patients. These are the exceptions to the rule, those with bowels that move too often (more than 3 times a day.) This includes those with Colitis, Irritable Bowel Syndrome, Crohn's Disease, etc. If your bowels are irritated, inflamed, hot or working too frequently, skip this formula and go directly to **Intestinal Formula #2.**

For price and quantity information please refer to your American Botanical Pharmacy 2001 Herbal Product Catalog or call 1-800-HERBDOC for your FREE copy.

DR. SCHULZE'S INTESTINAL FORMULA #2

BOTANICAL INGREDIENTS *Flax seed,* Linum usitatissimum, **Apple Fruit Pectin,** *Malus communis,* **Pharmaceutical Grade Bentonite Clay, Psyllium seed and husk,** *Plantago ovata,* **Slippery Elm inner Bark,** *Ulmus fulva,* **Marshmallow root,** *Althaea officinalis,* **Peppermint leaf,** *Mentha piperita* and **Activated Willow Charcoal,** *Salix alba.*

METABOLIC ACTION AND BOTANICAL CHEMISTRY This formula contains the three most powerful and effective absorbers and neutralizers known, Clay, Charcoal and Pectin. Our **Pharmaceutical Grade Bentonite Clay** is the most powerful, coming from the high desert and naturally dried so it contains no gas residues. It is a non-specific drawing agent, a powerful vacuum that literally removes everything. It will literally absorb up to 40 times its weight in intestinal fecal matter and waste. This bentonite clay also smothers and draws out intestinal parasites. The **Activated Willow Charcoal** is the greatest absorbing agent for every toxin and poison known. This is why you find charcoal inside every water filter. Our willow charcoal will absorb and render harmless over 3,000 known drug residues, pesticides, insecticides and just about every harmful chemical known. **Apple Fruit Pectin** is highly osmotic and literally draws numerous harmful substances out of your intestines, especially heavy metals like mercury and lead, even carcinogenic radioactive materials like strontium 90.

This formula also contains four of the most soothing and demulcent herbs known for the intestinal mucosa (the lining of the colon). These herbs are Flax seed, Psyllium seed, Slippery Elm bark and Marshmallow root. **Flax seed** is an oil seed and these oils are protective to the colon lining. Rich in omega 3 and 6 Essential Fatty Acids and oils, these EFA's are highly soothing and anti-inflammatory to the intestinal wall and are a natural laxative. It also is a great softening agent and helps to liquefy old, hardened fecal matter for easy removal. **Psyllium seed and husks** are so effective, they are listed in almost every major medical text as a treatment for irritable bowel. Psyllium is highly anti-inflammatory and also normalizes bowel action. While it will ease diarrhea and slow the passage time of fecal contents by bonding with the water, it also relieves constipation and speeds up the passage of fecal matter by increasing and bulking up the volume of the stool. **Slippery Elm inner bark** is highly mucilaginous. When mixed with liquid it produces a soothing and slippery paste that coats and protects the bowel, reduces inflammation and absorbs excess acid. **Marshmallow root** has been used for centuries in Traditional European Medicine to alleviate intestinal irritation. These four herbs working together create an incredible soothing coating anti-inflammatory paste that clings to the lining of the colon.

Finally, **Peppermint leaf** is added to this formula for a few reasons. First, it is highly anti-spasmodic to the entire digestive tract, reducing spasms and reducing the pain caused by them. Secondly, it is carminative in action, reducing, relieving and moving gas. Gas can be created when doing any deep bowel cleansing because intestinal and gastric fluids react with old, putrid fecal matter that is being lifted off the walls of the colon.

DOSAGE

Before beginning **Intestinal Formula #2**, your bowels should be moving at least three times a day, or at least once for each meal you eat. Continue using Intestinal Formula #1 until this is achieved.

Take Intestinal Formula #2 five times a day. Mix one heaping teaspoon of the powder with 8 ounces of juice or distilled water in a jar with a lid. Shake it vigorously and drink it immediately. Take it anytime during the day. Just be sure to allow about 30 minutes before or after meals, juices or taking your tinctures. Use the entire 8 ounce jar in one week.

HELPFUL HINT: Put a small amount of water in your jar first. Add the powder and then shake it. Then add more water. This keeps the powder from sticking to the jar, making it easier to clean.

This formula contains bentonite clay and may be binding. Patient Type A may need to increase dosage by one capsule of Intestinal Formula #1. Patient Type B may need to take one Intestinal Formula #1 in the evening if you find you are a little constipated.

For price and quantity information please refer to your American Botanical Pharmacy 2001 Herbal Product Catalog or call 1-800-HERBDOC for your FREE copy.

DR. SCHULZE'S INTESTINAL FORMULA #3

BOTANICAL INGREDIENTS *Senna leaf and pod, Cassia angustifolia,* **Cascara Sagrada aged bark,** *Rhamnus purshiana,* **Anise seed,** *Pimpinella anisum,* **Clove bud,** *Syzgium aromaticum,* **Tangerine oil,** *Citrus reticulata,* and **California Fig concentrate,** *Caricae fructus.*

METABOLIC ACTION AND BOTANICAL CHEMISTRY As stated under Intestinal Formula #1, **Senna leaf and pod** and **Cascara Sagrada aged bark** both contain the phytochemical anthraquinone, called emodin, which increases the normal muscular contractions (peristalsis) of the gastro-intestinal tract, especially the colon. This formula promotes soft, easy bowel movements and it will help strengthen the colon for better future elimination. Figs and prunes have been used effectively as a natural treatment for constipation since the beginning of recorded medical history. The base of this tonic, **California Fig concentrate,** acts not only as a mild natural laxative, but also make the formula sweet and tastes good for the kids. **Anise seed oil** and **Clove bud oil** are strong carminatives and antispasmodics and therefore are used to relieve gas, cramps, colic, indigestion, nausea and stomach aches. **Tangerine oil** is anti-bacterial but is also used to mask and flavor the medication.

DOSAGE

For adults:
(Generally if you need over 2 teaspoons then use Intestinal Formula #1.)
For children:

10 to 25 pounds	1/8 to 1/4 teaspoon	75 to 100 pounds	3/4 to 1 teaspoon
25 to 50 pounds	1/4 to 1/2 teaspoon	100 to 150 pounds	1 to 1 1/2 teaspoons
50 to 75 pounds	1/2 to 3/4 teaspoon	above 150 pounds	2 or more teaspoons

Kids love the taste, a sweet fig-tangerine flavor, so don't let them drink the whole bottle. Always start the children out with the lower dosages and work your way up to whatever dosage is needed. It is better to have them be constipated one more day than to have cramps, diarrhea or a pooping accident from taking too much, which can turn them off from ever using the formula again (and live a life of constipation). So take it easy on the dosage at first.

And of course, you may exceed dosages recommended above – whatever it takes to get the bowels working regularly.

For price and quantity information please refer to your American Botanical Pharmacy 2001 Herbal Product Catalog or call 1-800-HERBDOC for your FREE copy.

DR. SCHULZE'S DIGESTIVE FORMULA

BOTANICAL INGREDIENTS *Ginger rhizome, Zingiber officinale, Sweet Fennel seed, Foeniculum officinale, Peppermint leaf and Peppermint essential oil, Mentha piperita.*

METABOLIC ACTION AND BOTANICAL CHEMISTRY In this formula I combined three of the most effective and powerful carminative herbs, Jamaican Ginger rhizome, Sweet Fennel seed and Peppermint leaf and essential oil. **These three herbs make a powerful tonic that relieves gas, cramps, colic, bloating, heartburn, indigestion, nausea and pain in the digestive tract, especially the stomach.** This is the greatest formula for anyone who has any digestive problem. **Ginger rhizome, Sweet Fennel seed** and **Peppermint leaf** all contain essential oils that, according to medical texts and even the Merck Index, are therapeutically carminative. Ginger is also noted as an anti-emetic (against nausea), and peppermint as a gastric sedative and antispasmodic.

DOSAGE

Put 1 to 2 droppersful into 1 to 2 ounces of water and drink. Use as often as needed.

For price and quantity information please refer to your American Botanical Pharmacy 2001 Herbal Product Catalog or call 1-800-HERBDOC for your FREE copy.

DR. SCHULZE'S CAYENNE TINCTURE AND POWDER

BOTANICAL INGREDIENTS *Dr. Schulze's amazing special blend of the Fresh juice of Habanero peppers and dried Florida Habanero, California Jalapeno, African Birdseye, Chinese Bird, Thai Red, Korean Aji and Japanese species, but all grown in the United States. Capsicum species.*
NOTE: *The powder does not contain the Habanero juice.*

METABOLIC ACTION AND BOTANICAL CHEMISTRY Cayenne is the greatest herbal aid to circulation and can be used on a regular basis. There is no other herb that stimulates the blood flow so rapidly, powerfully and completely. After all, no other herbs give you a red face, that's blood! For emergency use, it is almost unlimited. It has been used for everything from heart attacks, strokes, fainting and shock to internal and external bleeding and arthritic pain and inflammation. This herb, in history, has been so revered by so many herbalists, some added it to almost every formulation, and I am one of them.

All hot Capsicum species contain the powerful phytochemicals capsaicin and oleoresins which are thought to be the active constituents.

DOSAGE

TINCTURE: 5 or more drops. CAUTION – it is EXTREMELY HOT. In an emergency situation, you can actually use droppersful.

POWDER: A small pinch added to drinks or food, CAUTION – it is EXTREMELY HOT. CAUTION – start with only a small amount! Do not encapsulate. This can be too shocking to the stomach and digestion. Put a small amount in a little juice, stir and chug. Work your way up in dosage slowly. 1/8 to 1/4 teaspoon two to four times daily.

<u>WARNING:</u> *This product contains extremely HOT Cayenne pepper. Wash hands two or three times after handling this product. Do not touch sensitive areas of the body after handling this powder. When we mix this Capsicum powder, even some of our employees who are used to consuming hot peppers have to wear special anti-contamination suits with special forces gas masks I bought in Germany. I am not joking.*

For price and quantity information please refer to your American Botanical Pharmacy 2001 Herbal Product Catalog or call 1-800-HERBDOC for your FREE copy.

CHAPTER 3

THE LIVER AND GALLBLADDER

EXPLANATION OF SYSTEM

THE LIVER

Although your medical doctor would like you to believe that they have figured your liver out and *got it all down,* the reality is that **your liver is the most metabolically complex organ in the entire human body**, more than even your brain. It has numerous different microscopic functional units and is as complex and infinite as outer space. One of the main reasons I know God was a natural healer and NOT a medical doctor is the liver itself. It is so incredibly complex you know it's best to just leave it alone and create a healing lifestyle for it, and DON'T TOUCH IT. HANDS OFF. Now, let me try to boil it down and make understanding the functions of the liver as simple as possible.

Your liver is the largest organ inside your body. It weighs around three pounds. It is on your right side under your lower ribs. The underneath of your liver is concave because it covers your stomach, duodenum, hepatic flexure of the colon, right kidney and right adrenal. Blood passes through your liver, especially blood from your digestive organs, which contain end products of digestion and nutrition, before this blood enters your general circulation to the rest of your body. If I were to divide the two main tasks of your liver they would be ENERGY & NUTRITION, and DETOXIFICATION.

ENERGY and NUTRITION

Your Liver is your Life Force, the source for your ENERGY. Your liver synthesizes the sugar glucose from carbohydrates or starches that you eat. Glucose is the most important carbohydrate in your body's metabolism. It could be called *PURE ENERGY* because it is used by your brain and every other cell of the body for just that--ENERGY. Excess glucose is stored in your liver as glycogen and is ready to be converted back to Glucose if any energy is needed. Your liver also stores other SUPER ENERGY NUTRIENTS like Vitamin B-12 and Iron to be used any time you need a turbo charge.

Your liver also makes vitamins, clotting factors and amino acids. It makes cholesterol that you need to produce steroid hormones (sex hormones) and other important metabolic chemicals. It also makes the lipoproteins like HDLs that transport fat around in your blood. *(Too much cholesterol in your blood, causing coronary arterial blockages, is from eating too much animal food and rarely from a liver gone haywire.)* The liver stores other vitamins too, like A, D, E and K.

DETOXIFICATION

Your Liver is THE blood detoxification organ of your body. The liver recycles and removes worn out blood cells.

Each red blood cell has a life span of 120 days (4 months). Once it is old and its time is up, Macrophages (*big eating* white blood cells in your liver) eat the red blood cell. Every RBC (*red blood cell*) contains Hemoglobin. Hemoglobin is the iron containing pigment in your blood that makes it red, which carries the oxygen from your lungs to all the cells of your body. Your liver recycles this iron, stores it for later use or turns it into bile, which it excretes as a digestive juice. **Bile stimulates digestion, emulsifies fats, stimulates peristalsis (the muscular waves of the intestines), is a natural laxative and a natural digestive antiseptic.** Bile contains bilirubin, a yellow-orange pigment from the iron in the hemoglobin from the dead red blood cells that macrophages ate phew…, if you didn't catch that one don't worry. Remember, getting well is easy.

Now for you numbers freaks. Each red blood cell has over 200 million hemoglobin molecules in it and you have over 35 trillion red blood cells, so that's over 7,000,000,000,000,000 *(How the heck do you say this number?)* hemoglobin molecules that your liver has to recycle or over 58,000,000,000,000 *(58 trillion)* hemoglobin molecules every day.

OK let's get simple. The liver detoxifies, metabolizes, renders harmless and eliminates harmful toxic poisons, chemicals and substances from your blood. It produces many different enzymes that actually convert toxic poisons into harmless chemicals which are eliminated in the bile that your liver excretes.

A small list of the substances that your liver detoxifies and renders harmless are alcoholic drinks, street drugs, pharmaceutical drugs, insecticides, pesticides, food additives, environmental toxic chemicals, parasites, bacteria and virus. **So one of the liver's main jobs is to eliminate toxins, chemicals, poisons and drugs from your body. Then it only makes sense that the more intake you have of toxic substances, the harder it is on your liver, the more work it has to do.** This makes a great case for organic food. It not only tastes better and is more nutritious, but it doesn't overwork or deplete your liver.

The liver also has to metabolize and render harmless anything that causes increased ammonia in the body. The main culprit here is animal food. When animal food is digested it forms ammonia, an alkaline gas, which is absorbed by your intestines into your blood hopefully to be converted into urea by your liver to be removed by your kidneys. Americans being the highest consumers of animal food on the planet per person, have a constant over production of ammonia gas in the intestines which in turn weakens the liver and promotes hepatic coma or paralysis of the liver. Substances that contain ammonia, besides animal flesh, organs, eggs and milk, are mainly drugs such as sedatives, tranquilizers, anesthetics, analgesics (pain relievers) and diuretics. **(AT HOME EXPERIMENT: Take two aspirin and place them in a spoon. Hold the spoon over a candle or the stove until the aspirin melt. WOW, ammonia city.)** For years in my clinic I saw patient after patient with liver trauma and even acute failure that caused hepatic coma worse than alcohol, drugs and toxic poisons. **IT WAS CAUSED BY HIGH PROTEIN FAD DIETS.** These diets have come and gone. The current ones are the Zone and Atkins. These diets, like any diet, can cause weight loss, but they can also skyrocket your ammonia levels and paralyze your liver. This is a double whammy because your liver now cannot process all of this added cholesterol that you are eating more and more of, and this alone could give you a heart attack or stroke. Granted you will look fit and trim in the hospital bed or the casket, but better to have a healthy liver than to be sick or dead.

JAUNDICE: When your Liver Gets Sick

As I have discussed, one of the liver's primary jobs is the production of bile, which is its waste product and also a great digestive system aid among many other things. When the liver gets sick, it gets constipated and the bile instead of getting released, **backs up in the body.** Remember the part about the 58 trillion hemoglobin molecules that the liver has to process EVERY DAY from the dead red blood cells? Well, when the liver backs up with bile which contains bilirubin (an **orange-red** iron pigment from the old hemoglobin that the liver eats) and at the same time the liver can't continue to clean all the 58 trillion dead **orange-red** hemoglobin molecules out of your blood, in a very short time you have all this excess circulating **orange-red** bilirubin and hemoglobin and what color do you think you are going to turn? You guessed it, <u>ORANGE-RED.</u> When your sclera (the whites of your eyes), your skin and even your urine takes on an orange-red color, this is called jaundice and <u>**is a good sign that your liver is very constipated, it is that simple. This is why one of the major cleansing and detoxifying aids I used in my clinic was a liver flush, to unconstipate the liver and get the bile flowing again.**</u> There are two main types of jaundice and they are referred to as Intra Hepatic (inside your liver) and Extra Hepatic (outside of your liver) referring to where it is thought the trouble is.

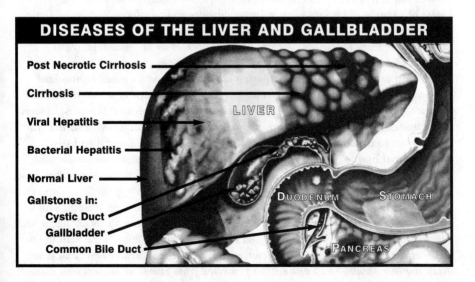

DISEASES OF THE LIVER AND GALLBLADDER

- Post Necrotic Cirrhosis
- Cirrhosis
- Viral Hepatitis
- Bacterial Hepatitis
- Normal Liver
- Gallstones in:
    - Cystic Duct
    - Gallbladder
    - Common Bile Duct

LIVER

DUODENUM   STOMACH

PANCREAS

INTRA HEPATIC JAUNDICE

The most common causes of Hepatitis (*which just means liver inflammation*) and Intra Hepatic Jaundice are drugs, alcohol, liver damage, almost any virus, bacteria, fungus, fad heavy animal protein weight loss diets and viral hepatitis.

VIRAL HEPATITIS

There are currently 6 known types of viral hepatitis. The most commonly known are Hepatitis A, Hepatitis B and what used to be referred to as Hepatitis non-A, non-B which is now called Hepatitis C, and Hepatitis D, E and G. Soon we will discover so many more that we will run out of letters of the alphabet and have to start giving them names like tropical storms and hurricanes, like Hepatitis Harry. There is currently a medical mass panic to vaccinate for Hepatitis C. This dangerous vaccination is even given to children born in hospitals in NYC within hours after birth and most school kids in California. But the only real prevention is to STOP doing what hurts your liver – like drugs and toxins – and START living a healthy liver lifestyle. As I said earlier, the liver's job is to neutralize poisons and toxins and the more a person or child is bombarded with poisons, the weaker the liver becomes. What poisons, you ask? Well when was the last time you were around a typical American kid and watched him eat? Or any adult for that matter? Weak livers have less resistance to infections. We will never get rid of germs and viruses. As I always say, the only defense is a strong offense building a strong healthy body. The massive amount of hepatitis infections all around America is just a reflection that we have beaten up our livers for too long.

EXTRA HEPATIC JAUNDICE

The most common cause of extra hepatic jaundice is some type of blockage. Sounds like my theory of all diseases being caused by blockage, doesn't it? And the major blockage is gall stones stuck in the gallbladder and bile ducts. Remember I said earlier that over a half million people this year in America will have their gallbladders carved out of them by medical doctors. Medical doctors are so absolutely stupid. **FLUSH IT OUT. Don't CUT IT OUT.**

Minor jaundice or liver constipation can go on for years almost unnoticed causing all sort of health related problems. Neurological diseases, neuromuscular diseases, paralysis, chronic fatigue, immune system depression and disorders, cancers, heart disease, stroke, hypertension, high cholesterol, every digestive disorder from indigestion to constipation, diabetes, dementia, depression, painful and stiff joints, sexual dysfunction, eyesight problems, the list is almost endlesssssssssss.

Many old sage doctors used to say when you have someone that has cancer, you have a patient who had a sick liver three to five years ago. I will go a step further. With any sick patient and with any disease, we need to look at the liver and get it clean. This is why in my clinic, EVERYONE, EVERY PATIENT, had to do my 5 Day Cleansing and Detoxification Program and my Liver and Gallbladder Flush. What is the bottom line?

Let the liver get run down and congested and you will become toxic and weak. Keep the liver healthy and you will be protected from chemical poisons and disease. You'll feel great and have TONS of energy.

THE GALLBLADDER

The gallbladder is a pear shaped sac on the underside of the right lobe of the liver that stores bile from the liver. While in the gallbladder the bile is concentrated by removing water. The bile is released through the cystic duct, which joins the hepatic duct from the liver to create the common bile duct which empties into the duodenum (the beginning of the small intestine, see picture on page 10.) Bile is not only the waste product of the liver that carries away the neutralized poisons, but as stated previously, also stimulates digestion, aids digestion by emulsifying fats, stimulates peristalsis (the muscular waves of the intestines), is a natural laxative and a natural digestive antiseptic.

When the bile contains too much cholesterol from eating too much animal food (or for some people ANY animal food) the cholesterol can't be kept in solution anymore and forms quite hard stones and rocks. These can form in the gallbladder and also the bile ducts causing extra hepatic jaundice.

GLOSSARY OF LIVER AND GALLBLADDER TERMINOLOGY

Bile   thick bitter-tasting fluid secreted by the liver. Bile aids in the digestion of fat, and also stimulates peristalsis, acting as a natural laxative. Bile contains cholesterol, lecithin, and mucin as well as bile pigments which are responsible for the variety of colors observed in it. Some of the pigments are breakdown products of the hemoglobin in red blood cells that have died. The liver breaks down red blood cells recycling some of the components to be used to make new red blood cells. The red pigment in red blood cells breaks down to yellow, green, blue, orange and brown. Bilirubin is the brown pigment responsible for the brown appearance of feces.

Bili   pertaining to the bile. Biliary colic – "a gallbladder attack"

Cirrhosis   end-stage degeneration of the liver which usually results from a long-standing injury to the liver as in chronic alcoholism or chronic hepatitis. The liver shrinks and becomes filled with scar tissue and fat, making it difficult for blood to pass through the liver. The symptoms are bleeding tendency, collection of fluid in the abdomen, jaundice, reddening of the palms, itching, indigestion, constipation or diarrhea, and can lead to serious mental abnormalities.

Gallstone   stone that forms in the gallbladder, most often made of cholesterol covered by a calcium shell that causes pain when it passes out of the gallbladder and gets stuck in the narrow bile duct; can also be made of broken down red blood cells, especially in the case of certain anemias

Hepato   pertaining to the liver

Hepatitis   inflammation of the liver usually caused by a virus. Different types are A, B, C, and E. Chronic hepatitis B and C over the years can turn into liver cancer or cirrhosis.

Hepatocarcinoma liver cancer

Interferon   drug that mimics the effects of interferon made naturally in the body. Interferon stops viral infections from spreading. It is used as a treatment for hepatitis, and has a low success rate.

Jaundice   yellowish discoloration of the skin, the whites of the eyes, and other tissues due to excess circulating bilirubin; usually caused by a blockage in the liver (by stones, cancer or scar tissue), an infection of the liver or by hemolytic anemia

Liver transplant procedure during which a surgeon removes the patient's liver and replaces it with the liver of someone else; usually performed when the liver is failing as in cirrhosis of the liver or end stage hepatitis.

SPECIFIC HERBAL FORMULAE
FOR THE LIVER & GALLBLADDER

DR. SCHULZE'S LIVER/GALLBLADDER & ANTI-PARASITE FORMULA

BOTANICAL INGREDIENTS *Milk Thistle seed,* Silybum marianum, **Dandelion root,** Taraxacum officinale, **Oregon Grape root,** Berberis aquifolium, **Gentian root,** Gentiana lutea, **Wormwood leaf and flower,** Artemisia Absinthium, **Mojave Chaparral herb,** Larrea californica, **Black Walnut hulls,** Juglans nigra, **Ginger rhizome,** Zingiber officinale, **Garlic bulb,** Allium sativum, **and Fennel seed,** Foeniculum officinale.

METABOLIC ACTION AND BOTANICAL CHEMISTRY The herbs in this formula are famous for their ability to stimulate, cleanse and protect the liver and gallbladder and rid the body of parasites. **Milk Thistle** contains many phytochemicals, three chief ones being silibinin, silydianin and silychristin. These 3 plant chemicals are often collectively referred to as *silymarin*. There are many ways in which these plant chemicals protect and heal your liver – too many for this book. But two main ones are **protection** and **regeneration**. **The phytochemicals in Milk Thistle actually strengthen the structure of the hepatocytes (liver cells), skin or membrane which prevents the penetration of known liver toxins.**

These protective chemicals also stimulate the action of the nucleolar polymerase A, resulting in an increase in ribosomal protein synthesis and thus stimulate the regeneration of damaged liver cells and stimulate the formation of new liver cells. These chemicals are so powerful they can even protect you from some of the most lethal poisons on the planet, like death-cap mushrooms. Simply put, ingesting Milk thistle is like putting a protective coating around your current liver cells while it also speeds repair of damaged ones and builds new strong ones.

Oregon Grape rootbark, Gentian root, Wormwood leaves and **Dandelion root** are some of the most bitter plants on the planet and all classic bitter liver tonic herbs. They contain phytochemicals like berberine alkaloids and volatile oils which stimulate the liver to produce more bile which will flush out the bile ducts and gallbladder.

The **Black Walnut hulls, Wormwood** and **Garlic** are strong ANTI-PARASITICAL plants. Parasite infestation is a fact of life. One cubic inch of choice beef can have over 1,000 living parasite larvae waiting to hatch in your body. Over 65% of fresh fish tested had toxic levels of bacteria and parasites. Chicken is even worse. I've had hundreds of patients expel toilet bowls full of intestinal parasites, including tape worms over 30 FEET LONG. They have also killed cellular parasites with this formula. It works best if used in conjunction with both Intestinal Formulas #1 and #2. Use if parasites are suspected, or if there has been a history of bowel problems, constipation, eating of animal products, prolonged illness, disease and degeneration. If you have been exposed to any toxic substances, or drank alcohol or other harmful beverages, this formula is for you. It is also beneficial if you have had high cholesterol, blood fats or any family history of liver or gallbladder problems. Many believe that anyone who has cancer or any immune dysfunction had a weak congested liver to begin with. Even if a person had their gallbladder removed, these herbs will still be effective in cleaning the liver and bile ducts.

DOSAGE

2 droppersful (60 drops) three to four times daily for 1 week. This formula is most effective if used in conjunction with the Detoxification Tea and also my 5 Day Cleansing and Detoxification Program with the Liver/Gallbladder Flush.

For price and quantity information please refer to your American Botanical Pharmacy 2001 Herbal Product Catalog or call 1-800-HERBDOC for your FREE copy.

DR. SCHULZE'S DETOXIFICATION TEA

BOTANICAL INGREDIENTS *Dandelion root, Taraxacum officinale,* **Burdock root,** *Arctium lappa,* **Cardamon seed,** *Elettaria cardamomum,* **Ginger root,** *Zingiber officinale,* **Pau d'Arco bark,** *Tahebubia impetigenosa,* **Clove bud,** *Syzgium aromaticum,* **Fennel seed,** *Foeniculum officinale,* **Licorice root,** *Glycyrrhiza glabra,* **Juniper berries,** *Juniperus communis,* **Black Peppercorns,** *Piper nigrum,* **Uva Ursi leaf,** *Arctostaphylos uva ursi,* **Horsetail herb,** *Equisetum arvense,* **Parsley root,** *Petroselinium crispum, and* **Orange Peel,** *Citrus species, and* **Cinnamon bark,** *Cinnamomum cassia.*

METABOLIC ACTION AND BOTANICAL CHEMISTRY Ginger root, Cardamon seed, Fennel seed, Cinnamon bark, Black Peppercorns and Clove bud are famous classic digestive herbs. They are extremely effective and have been a part of traditional Chinese, Indian, European and American herbal medicine for centuries. They are specifics for dyspepsia (basically gas), cramps, colic, bloating, indigestion, heartburn, and nausea. They contain essential oils which stimulate ALL aspects of digestion from saliva excretion and digestive juice stimulation to antispasmodic and even stimulate the villi of the small intestine for better assimilation.

Cardamon seeds, Roasted Dandelion root, Burdock root and Orange Peel all stimulate the liver to excrete more bile. While Cardamon has essential oils that cause this hepatic action the three latter herbs all contain bitter hepatic stimulating phytochemicals. Dandelion and Burdock also stimulate the kidneys to excrete more urine along with the **Horsetail herb** and **Parsley root. Juniper berries** and **Uva Ursi leaf** are also diuretics and urinary tract disinfectants. They make you urinate more and destroy urinary infections (See Kidney/Bladder Formula, Chapter 4). **Pau d'Arco inner-bark** is a classic South American immune stimulant and **Licorice root** is soothing and healing to the lining of the entire digestive tract.

DOSAGE

<u>General Cleansing and Detoxification:</u> 2 cups of Detoxification Tea three times per day.

<u>Directions for making the Tea:</u> Put 6 tablespoons of Detoxification Tea into 60 ounces of distilled water. Be sure to use only stainless steel or glass cookware. Let the tea sit in the water overnight. In the morning heat to a boil, reduce heat and simmer for 15 minutes. Strain the herbs. Do not discard them. Let the tea cool a bit, but use it hot. This will give you enough tea for your 6 cups for the day. Put the used herbs back into the pot, add 3 tablespoons of fresh herbs and 60 ounces of distilled water. Let sit overnight and repeat the whole process. Keep adding new herbs to old ones for three days; then discard all herbs and start over.

<u>For a Coffee Replacement:</u> Make as needed, using 1-2 tablespoons of tea in 20 ounces of distilled water. Bring to a boil; reduce heat and simmer for 15 minutes. Drink the tea hot.

CHAPTER 4

THE KIDNEYS, BLADDER AND URINARY TRACT

EXPLANATION OF SYSTEM

Very simply put, **the Urinary System is comprised of two Kidneys, one Bladder and a series of tubes.** The Kidneys look similar to Kidney beans in shape and also have a similar purple-brown color. They each weigh about 5 ounces and are about the same size as the palm of your hand not including your fingers or thumb. You have one on each side of your spine. The top of each Kidney is about at the 12th Thoracic vertebra and the bottom being about at the 3rd Lumbar vertebra, (from your mid to lower back). They are almost completely covered by your lowest back ribs.

The inner side (spinal side) of each Kidney has an indentation, the smaller curve of the Kidney shape, which is called the **hilus** or **hilum.** This is where all the tubes that take blood in and out, and urine out of your Kidneys connect and go into the Kidney, these being the **renal** (_renalis_ is Latin for Kidney) **artery**, the **renal vein** and the **ureter**. **The Renal Artery brings blood to the Kidney to be filtered and cleaned. The Renal Vein returns clean blood back to your body and the waste liquid, urine, leaves the Kidney via the Ureter. Both Ureters from each Kidney connect to the Bladder.** As with all metabolic processes of the human body, this process of blood filtering and urine formation is also very intricate, detailed, complex. In other words, beyond mankind's comprehension. Knowing that, I will simplify this process so you have a basic understanding of what the Kidneys do and how they do it.

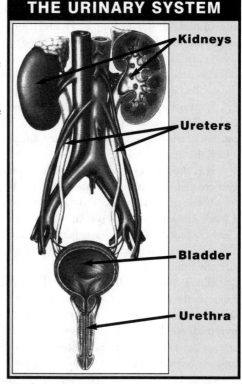

THE URINARY SYSTEM

Kidneys

Ureters

Bladder

Urethra

Each Kidney is divided into between 8 and 18 wedge shaped chambers called **renal pyramids**. Each of these pyramids contains the many parts of the Kidney that come into play for the blood to be filtered. The outside of each **renal pyramid** is called the **renal cortex** (cortex is Latin for *rind* or *outer edge*), and the inside closest to the **hilus** or smaller curve of the Kidney is called the **renal medulla** (medulla is Latin for *inner* or *center*).

THE KIDNEY

Renal (Kidney) Pyramids (each pyramid contains 50,000 to 125,000 nephrons)

Renal Artery

Ureter

The **renal artery** branches off inside the Kidney to form numerous smaller arteries which enter the outer portion of the Kidney, the **renal cortex**. A very small renal artery branch eventually enters one of the many **Nephrons** (now that you know the Latin for Kidney, *renalis* hence renal, *nephros* is Greek for Kidney).

The Nephrons are the individual small filtering units in your Kidney and it is believed that each Kidney contains approximately one million of these Nephrons.

Inside each **Nephron** is a **renal corpuscle** and a **renal tubule**. The renal corpuscle is made up of a capillary network called a **glomerulus** enclosed in a **Bowman's capsule**. The **renal tubule** extends from the **Bowman's capsule** via the **proximal convoluted tubule**, the **loop of Henle,** the **distal convoluted tubule** and the **collecting tubule** all of which are surrounded and wrapped by **peritubular capillaries.** [Note: capillaries, from the Latin *capillaris* meaning *hair-like*, are the smallest of the blood vessels/tubes, averaging 0.008mm in diameter which connect the very ends of the smallest arteries (arterioles) to the beginnings of the smallest veins (venules).]

Eventually the filtered blood waste (urine) enters into **collecting tubules** and then eventually the **papillary ducts** which are in the **renal medulla** or the inner or center portion of the Kidney. These **papillary ducts** eventually empty into the **ureter** through which the urine leaves the Kidney.

It is the Kidneys' job to filter blood plasma, return good blood to the body and create urine to carry waste out of the body.

While many know that most cars have water cooled engines, the human Kidney is a water run waste removal system. Much of the water that you consume is necessary to clean the blood and flush waste material out of the body via the Kidneys. The Kidneys also regulate the water, electrolyte and acid/alkaline balance of the blood and indirectly, all body fluids.

Blood enters your Kidneys in the inner indented section **(hilus)** closest to the spine via the **renal artery.** Inside your Kidney this artery divides into many other smaller arteries that enter one of the pyramid shaped separate kidney chambers **(renal pyramid)** and branch into even smaller arteries in the **renal cortex**. One of these small arteries enters a very small microscopic sac **(nephron)** which is an individual filtering unit. As blood passes inside the **nephron** into the **renal corpuscle** through the

glomerulus and **Bowman's capsule,** water and dissolved substances and small bits are filtered out of the blood but big things like blood cells and large proteins are retained in the **capillaries** and blood. As the water and dissolved substances that were filtered out of the blood which is now called **glomerular filtrate** (we could call this pre-pee) passes through the **renal tubules,** the **proximal convoluted tubule,** the **loop of Henle,** the **distal convoluted tubule** and the **collecting tubule,** it moves into the other area of the Kidney called the **renal medulla.** Here the urine goes into the **papillary ducts** and eventually leaves the Kidneys through the **ureter.**

Useful materials such as water, glucose, amino acids, vitamins and minerals are reabsorbed into the blood via the small **capillaries.** This reabsorbtion is monitored and limited by your body. The reabsorbtion of nutrients is stopped if you have too much of a nutrient already and the reabsorbtion of water is regulated by hormones.

The Kidneys are the organ mainly responsible for not only the filtering of the blood, but by monitoring the acid-alkaline balance they also regulate the physical properties and composition of the blood. What is left in the remaining liquid that is now called urine is about 95% water and 5% dissolved substances. The dissolved substances are minerals, especially sodium, nitrogenous waste products like urea, uric acid, creatine, creatinine, ammonia, chlorides, calcium, magnesium, phosphorous and many other substances like blood, pus, bacteria, parasites, all depending on the disease or health level of the person.

The urine leaves each Kidney via the **ureter** and both right and left Kidney ureters connect to the Bladder separately, on the corresponding side. The Bladder is a general term from the Anglo-Saxon *blaedre* meaning a sac or receptacle for a secretion, like the Gallbladder. The **urinary bladder** then, of course, is the muscular receptacle for urine, and without it your urine would just constantly run out of your body. The Bladder is in the lower front of your pelvic cavity. In women it is in front of the vagina and in men in front of the rectum.

The Bladder has a normal storage capacity of about a quart or more. When the Bladder fills, it stretches, which initiates nerve impulses to the spinal cord. When you want to urinate, returning motor nerve impulses simultaneously cause contraction of the bladder and relaxation of the bladder sphincter muscle. This process can be stopped temporarily by the voluntary contraction of the external urethral sphincter muscle.

At the very bottom of the Bladder is the **urethra**, a tube that the urine passes through to leave the body. On the man this tube passes through the center of the prostate gland, through the center of the penis, and out the end. It is also used for the passage of semen. This is why when a man has a swollen prostate due to sexual dysfunction or disease, it squeezes off the urethra making voiding urine very difficult. In a woman, the urethra leaves the bladder and the orifice where the urine is voided is in the vestibule between the vagina and the clitoris.

GLOSSARY OF URINARY SYSTEM TERMINOLOGY

Anuria	no urine being produced
BPH	short for benign prostatic hypertrophy; an enlargement of the prostate gland causing a blockage of the urine flow through it. Symptoms include difficulty starting urine stream, decreased force of the urine stream and having to get up multiple times at night to urinate.
Cystitis	infection of the urinary bladder
Dialysis	process of diffusing blood across a semipermeable membrane to remove toxic materials and to maintain fluid, electrolyte, and acid-base balance in cases of impaired kidney function or absence of the kidneys. Usually, a patient is hooked up to a dialysis machine. Tubing runs from a vein to the machine and back again in a process called hemodialysis.
Glomerulo-nephritis	inflammation of the glomeruli of the kidney(s) causing blood and protein in the urine, swelling of the body, and high blood pressure
Hematuria	presence of blood in the urine
Hypertension	high blood pressure. Over the long-term, high blood pressure causes damage to the kidneys often to the point of kidney failure, making dialysis necessary.
Incontinence	inability to retain urine, semen, or feces due to loss of sphincter control or because of brain or spinal cord damage
Intravenous pyelogram	(IVP) – an X-ray of the pelvis of the kidney and the ureter in which a dye in injected intravenously. Multiple X-rays are taken while the patient is excreting the dye. The dye shows up white on a black background showing the structure of the kidneys and ureters. It is used to find blockages (especially kidney stones) and structural abnormalities of these organs.
Nephrotic Syndrome	a kidney disease marked by overall swelling of the body and high blood pressure
Nocturia	excessive urination during the night

Oliguria	urinating only a small amount; an abnormal condition
Polyuria	urinating excessively
Prostate	endocrine gland that surrounds the neck of the bladder and the urethra in the male. The gland secretes a thin fluid that forms part of the seminal fluid.
Pyelonephritis	infection of the kidney(s)
Renal	pertaining to the kidney(s)
Renal calculus	kidney stone. Types: calcium oxalate is the most common; uric acid – next common. The pain of a kidney stone lodged in a ureter is considered the worst pain you can have. Pain is either in the groin or in the kidney area. Stones can also cause blood in the urine.
Renal Cell Carcinoma	most common type of kidney cancer
Ureters	tubes that carry urine from the kidneys to the bladder
Urethra	the tube that carries urine from the bladder to the outside of the body
Urinalysis	an analysis of a urine specimen, usually ordered to test for infection, stones, cancer, and other urinary tract diseases

---

"Life is not a dress rehearsal. This is it, RIGHT NOW! You can choose to live it to the fullest or sit on the sidelines and watch it go by."

- Dr. Richard Schulze

SPECIFIC HERBAL FORMULAE FOR THE URINARY SYSTEM

DR. SCHULZE'S KIDNEY/BLADDER FORMULA

BOTANICAL INGREDIENTS *Uva Ursi leaf,* Arctostaphylos uva ursi, **Juniper berries,** Juniperus communis, **Corn silk,** Zea mays, **Horsetail herb,** Equisetum arvense, **Burdock root and seed,** Arctium lappa, **Parsley leaf and root,** Petroselinium crispum, **Pipsissewa leaf,** Chimaphilla umbellata **and Goldenrod flower tops,** Solidago virgaurea.

METABOLIC ACTION AND BOTANICAL CHEMISTRY Uva Ursi leaf contains powerful phytochemicals such as volatile oils, arbutin, quercetin, and mallic and gallic acids. Arbutin is highly antibacterial and destroys bacteria and fungus that infect the urinary system such as E. coli, Candida albicans, Staphylococcus, etc. One of the ways arbutin does this is by releasing aglycone hydroquinone and other phytochemicals into the urine. Quercetin is a capillary protectant, protecting the literally trillions of capillaries existing as part of the delicate kidney filtering system. Mallic and Gallic acids, the same as found in apples and apple cider vinegar have long been used for kidney and bladder infections.

All of the other herbs in this formula contain phytochemicals that are either diuretic, anti-microbial or anti-inflammatory to the entire urinary system.

DOSAGE
1-2 droppersful (30-60 drops) in a few ounces of water 3 to 4 times daily, depending on the diuretic action needed or the seriousness of the infection. Best results are obtained if used for 10 days or until the 2 ounce bottle is finished.

NOTE: *This formula is most effective when used in conjunction with the next formula, the Kidney/Bladder Tea and also Dr. Schulze's 5 Day Cleansing and Detoxification Program.*

For price and quantity information please refer to your American Botanical Pharmacy 2001 Herbal Product Catalog or call 1-800-HERBDOC for your FREE copy.

DR. SCHULZE'S KIDNEY/BLADDER HERB TEA

BOTANICAL INGREDIENTS *Juniper berries,* Juniperus communis, **Corn silk,** Zea mays, **Uva Ursi leaves,** Arctostaphylos uva ursi, **Parsley root and leaf,** Petroselinium crispum, **Carrot tops, Dandelion leaf,** Taraxacum officinale, **Horsetail herb,** Equisetum arvense, **Goldenrod flower tops,** Solidago virgaurea, **Hydrangea root,** Hydrangea arboresens, **Gravel root,** Eupatorium purpureum, **Marshmallow root,** Althea officinalis, **Orange peel,** Citrus species, **and Peppermint leaf,** Mentha piperita.

METABOLIC ACTION AND BOTANICAL CHEMISTRY The herbs in this formula have the identical action as the Kidney and Bladder Formula with the addition of **Hydrangea root** and **Gravel root** which are specifics for dissolving kidney stones and renal calculi.

Juniper berries are by far my favorite Kidney and Bladder herb. I used them in every clinical Kidney and Bladder Formula I ever made. I find them to be the diuretic herb that always works, and a urinary disinfectant that works even on the most stubborn cases. I believe this is due to their wonderful essential and volatile oils. They worked miracles in my clinic, but are not officially recognized for any of the above uses, but Uva Ursi is.

DOSAGE
2 cups three times daily.

<u>**Directions for making the tea:**</u> Put 6 tablespoons of this tea into 60 ounces of distilled water. Be sure to use only stainless steel or glass cookware. Let the tea sit in the water overnight. In the morning, heat it to a boil, reduce heat, and let simmer for 1 minute. Strain the herbs; do not discard them. Let the tea cool a bit, but use it hot. This will give you enough tea to drink 2 cups three times during the day. If you are planning to drink the tea for more than one day, then after the first day put the used herbs back into the pot, adding 3 tablespoons of fresh herbs and 60 ounces of distilled water. Let sit overnight and repeat the whole process. Keep adding new herbs to the old ones for three days, then discard all herbs and start all over.

NOTE: *This formula is most effective when used in conjunction with the previous formula, the Kidney/Bladder Formula and also Dr. Schulze's 5 Day Cleansing and Detoxification Program.*

For price and quantity information please refer to your American Botanical Pharmacy 2001 Herbal Product Catalog or call 1-800-HERBDOC for your FREE copy.

CHAPTER 5

THE HEART AND CIRCULATORY SYSTEM

EXPLANATION OF SYSTEM

Your heart is the muscular organ that contracts and relaxes rhythmically to pump blood throughout the body. It is located slightly to the left of the center of the chest touching the left and right lungs. It is a little larger than a fist.

The inside of the heart has four chambers – the left and right atria, and the left and right ventricles. The heart has four valves which make sure that blood does not flow backward in the wrong direction. The valve between the left atrium and left ventricle is the mitral valve. The valve between the right atrium and right ventricle is the tricuspid valve.

Although the main function of your heart is to carry oxygenated blood to all of the body, the heart itself needs the oxygen and nutrients from the blood, too. The heart pumps itself its own blood through the main outflow vessel, the aorta, and through the aorta to the coronary arteries to the actual heart muscle.

The blood circulates in the following manner. Blood enters the heart through two main vessels: the superior vena cava, a major vein which drains blood from the top half of the body, and the inferior vena cava. The inferior vena cava carries blood from the bottom half of the body to the heart. All blood enters into the right atrium of the heart. The right atrium contracts and sends the blood through the tricuspid valve to the right ventricle. The ventricles are the main pumping muscles. The right ventricle contracts and pumps the blood through the pulmonary arteries which lead to the lungs. When a person inhales, oxygen enters the lungs, and there the blood intermixes with the oxygen and carries it back to the heart through the pulmonary veins. Also, the carbon dioxide in the blood diffuses into the lungs and is eliminated from the body when a person exhales. The blood comes back to the left side of the heart now. It goes into the left atrium and is pumped through the mitral valve into the left ventricle. When blood fills the left ventricle, it contracts and pushes the blood through the aortic valve into the main artery of the body, the aorta. The ascending aorta ascends and branches off into smaller arteries (subclavian, carotid arteries, etc.) to supply blood to the top half of the body. Then, it descends (now it is called the descending aorta) and splits off into smaller arteries (the iliac, femoral arteries, etc.) to supply blood to the bottom half of the body. The arteries as they branch become smaller and smaller to become arterioles and finally capillaries that feed the cells on an individual level with oxygen and nutrients.

Tiny veins carry the blood back to the heart which is now oxygen-poor and contains carbon dioxide and waste products from the cells. The veins join to form larger veins until they become major veins like the inferior and superior vena cava that lead directly back to the heart. Now the cycle begins again. The time it takes to complete the entire cycle is about two minutes.

The heart is an electrical system. Heart muscle cells have the ability to generate spontaneous and rhythmic electric impulses on their own without any input from the nerves. (In fact, if a heart is maintained under proper conditions, it will continue to beat after removal from the body.) The electrical impulse begins in the sinoatrial node which is called the pacemaker because it sets the speed of the heartbeat. It conducts the impulse throughout the heart to the Bundle of His, the Purkinje fibers and the ventricular muscles, causing the heart to contract and relax rhythmically.

GLOSSARY OF CIRCULATORY SYSTEM TERMINOLOGY

Angina (pectoris) severe pain around the heart usually felt in the center of the chest, and sometimes radiating up to the neck and jaw or into the shoulder and down the left arm. It is sometimes accompanied by nausea and shortness of breath, and is caused by a shortage of blood to the heart from the coronary arteries. Attacks, aggravated by exercise or a stressful event, usually last less than 30 minutes and are relieved by rest or medication.

Angio pertaining to lymph or blood vessels; angioedema; angiogenesis

Angiogram (angio – blood vessel, gram – something written) an X-ray which shows the outlines of certain blood vessels. Angiography involves inserting an instrument into an artery (usually an artery in the leg) which is threaded up into the artery to be studied. Dye is injected into that artery and an X-ray is taken. The dye, which shows up black on the X-ray, shows the outlines of the artery lining, making cholesterol plaques visible. The rest of the picture shows white or faint gray.

Angioplasty balloon, etc.

Aneurysm localized abnormal bulging and weakening of a blood vessel wall, (usually an artery) that commonly enlarges and may rupture causing severe bleeding. Common causes are arteriosclerosis, infections of the arteries, inherited weakness in the wall, and trauma.

Arter-   pertaining to an artery; arteritis – inflammation of an artery

Arteriosclerosis   a disease of the arteries marked by thickening, hardening, and loss of elasticity in the arterial walls

Artery   blood vessel that carries oxygenated blood from the heart to the rest of the body

Athero-   fatty deposits, usually referring to those on the inside of arteries, as in atherosclerosis

Atherosclerosis   the buildup of cholesterol-lipid-calcium on the linings of the arteries. The cholesterol buildup eventually becomes a plaque which ulcerates, becomes calcified, and forms clots which may break off and travel to distant areas becoming lodged in smaller arteries (as in the coronary arteries, arteries in the eyes, kidney and brain).

Atrial Fibrillation   extremely rapid, incomplete contractions of the atria of the heart resulting in a rapid, irregular heartbeat. Often, blood stays in the atria and clots. The clots can break off and travel to the arteries of the brain causing a stroke.

Bicuspid Aortic Valve   the aortic valve has only two cusps (normally it has three). Because the structure is abnormal, the valve does not function perfectly and over time it calcifies and hardens, further worsening the valve's functions

Cardiomyopathy   disease of the heart muscle

Carotid endarterectomy   the surgical removal of the lining of the carotid artery in the neck; done when the artery has become blocked with cholesterol which causes strokes

Congestive Heart Failure   abbreviated as CHF. A failure of the heart muscle to pump the blood adequately. Usually the blood backs up into either the lungs (left-sided heart failure leading to an accumulation of fluid in the lungs), or in the abdomen (right-sided heart failure leading to swelling and fluid in the abdomen, liver, and legs.

Coronary artery disease   abbreviated as CAD.

Coronary Bypass Surgery	called a CABG for short (pronounced "cabbage") Open heart surgery during which leg veins are sewn on the heart, bypassing the clogged coronary arteries which can no longer supply oxygen to the heart
Endocardium	inner surface of the heart
Hypercholest-erolemia	too much cholesterol in the blood increasing risk for heart attack, stroke
Hypertension	high blood pressure
Ischemic Heart Disease	lack of oxygen supply to the heart usually caused by atherosclerosis of the coronary arteries (the coronary arteries get clogged with cholesterol)
Myocardium	the middle, or main muscular layer of the heart
Myocardial Infarction	commonly called an "MI"; means a heart attack. A portion of the myocardium dies due to lack of blood from blocked coronary arteries.
Myocarditis	inflammation of the heart muscle; usually caused by a virus
Pericarditis	inflammation of the outer sac surrounding the heart; usually occurs in association with an autoimmune disease like lupus or rheumatic heart disease
Rheumatic Heart Disease	infection of the heart valve(s), usually the mitral valve and aortic valve that follows a strep throat infection. It is caused by the streptococcus bacteria. The infection reoccurs periodically over years causing a gradual hardening and scarring of the heart valves, which can eventually lead to heart failure.
Sinoatrial Node	SA node for short; an area of the heart that signals the heart to beat. This signal is transmitted throughout the entire heart resulting in the contraction of the atria and ventricles which pumps the blood around the body.
Stroke	two types: hemorrhagic – a blood vessel in the brain bursts causing bleeding into the brain; ischemic – a blood clot lodges in a blood vessel in the brain, cutting off the blood supply to that part that depends on that blood vessel for oxygen. When this happens, that area of the brain is either "stunned" or dies. This is usually marked by a loss of consciousness followed by paralysis of the face and/or body. According to medical practitioners, only the "stunned" areas can recover if the blood vessel opens up again.

Ultrasonography use of ultrasound to produce an image or photograph of an organ or tissue. Ultrasound utilizes a certain frequency of inaudible sound waves that bounce off of tissues and record different signals for different densities of tissue. It is commonly used to evaluate the degree of blockage in an artery, commonly the carotid arteries, and leg arteries.

Vein blood vessel that carries oxygen-poor blood from the periphery of the body back to the heart. It has thinner, less muscular walls than an artery, and unlike an artery, contains valves which prevent the blood from flowing backward.

SPECIFIC HERBAL FORMULAE FOR THE CIRCULATORY SYSTEM

DR. SCHULZE'S HEART FORMULA

BOTANICAL INGREDIENTS *Hawthorne berry, flower and leaf, Crataegus oxycantha,* **Red Clover blossom,** *Trifolium pratense,* **Cactus grandiflorus stem and flower,** **Motherwort herb,** *Leonurus cardiaca,* **Garlic bulb,** *Allium sativum,* **Jamaican Ginger rhizome,** *Zingiber officinale,* **and Cayenne pepper,** *Capsicum annum.*

METABOLIC ACTION AND BOTANICAL CHEMISTRY **Hawthorne berry, flower** and **leaf** is a classic of Traditional European Medicine and has been used effectively for centuries for almost every type of heart and circulatory disease. It contains numerous potent phytochemicals including the flavonoids: hypercide, vitexinrhamnose, rutin, and vitexin and oligomeric procyanidins. These chemicals have been found in medical studies in America and abroad to have a direct effect on the heart, helping it to pump more easily, but with more force. They also help with the beta cells' conductivity from the nerve to muscle fibers, increase heart circulation, prevent stress related heart attacks, reduce angina pain and cardiac arrhythmia and are a potent cardiac boost for the elderly, giving them more energy.

In Asian medical studies it has been established that when Hawthorne is present in the blood, the heart muscle can function normally and survive on less blood and oxygen, as found in blocked coronary arteries. Also, if a heart attack does occur, the heart muscle can survive longer because the heart cells don't die as rapidly. It's also been established that if damage to the heart muscle does occur, it is much less in those who use Hawthorne than those who don't. For this reason I feel it is important for anyone with heart disease or a family history of heart disease to use this formula.

Red Clover blossom and **Garlic bulb.** These herbs have also proven themselves as potent and effective heart and circulatory medications, especially in thinning the blood which alleviates high blood pressure and reduces the risk of blood clots. Both of these actions reduce the risk of heart attack. Red Clover blossoms contain coumarins which inhibit the liver/vitamin K factor to reduce blood clots while Garlic's allicin reduces the red blood platelets from aggregating (sticking together). This is a great natural replacement for any heart patient who takes aspirin to thin the blood. Garlic is medically approved in most countries of the world as an effective treatment for hypertension and hypercholesterolemia, regulating blood pressure and lowering blood cholesterol, tryglyceride and fat levels.

Cactus grandiflorus stem contains cardiac glycosides almost identical to Digitalis lanata, the herb that the cardiac drug digitalis is made from. These glycosides increase the heart's pumping force without increasing the heart's oxygen demand, making the heart a more efficient pump and better able to meet the demands of the circulatory system. This makes it an excellent heart tonic and specific for congestive heart disease.

Motherwort herb is used throughout Europe and Asia as a general "fix all" cardiac tonic. It exhibits strong influence over the regularity of the heart beat, helping with both cardiac arrhythmia and taccycardia.

Last but not least, **Habanero pepper** and **Ginger rhizome** are the two best circulation stimulants known. Capsicum pepper species have been used as a remedy for heart attacks and strokes worldwide and have saved many lives. While Capsicum's influence seems to go to the heart first, Ginger goes to the extremities first and works backwards making them the dynamic duo for increasing the body's circulation.

DOSAGE

2 droppersful three to four times daily. This formula is a wonderful general heart and circulatory tonic. Best results occur when used continually over a long period of time. This formula is also most effective when used in conjunction with the **5 Day Cleansing and Detoxification Program** and the **Liver/Gallbladder Flush**, a zero cholesterol vegetarian food program, stress reduction and a moderate exercise routine.

For price and quantity information please refer to your American Botanical Pharmacy 2001 Herbal Product Catalog or call 1-800-HERBDOC for your FREE copy.

DR. SCHULZE'S CAYENNE TINCTURE AND POWDER

BOTANICAL INGREDIENTS *Dr. Schulze's amazing special blend of the Fresh juice of Habanero peppers and dried Florida Habanero, California Jalapeno, African Birdseye, Chinese Bird, Thai Red, Korean Aji and Japanese species, but all grown in the United States. Capsicum species.*
NOTE: *The powder does not contain the Habanero juice.*

METABOLIC ACTION AND BOTANICAL CHEMISTRY Cayenne is the greatest herbal aid to circulation and can be used on a regular basis. There is no other herb that stimulates the blood flow so rapidly, powerfully and completely. After all, no other herbs give you a red face, that's blood! For emergency use, it is almost unlimited. It has been used for everything from heart attacks, strokes, fainting and shock to internal and external bleeding and arthritic pain and inflammation. This herb, in history, has been so revered by so many herbalists, some added it to almost every formulation, and I am one of them.

All hot Capsicum species contain the powerful phytochemicals capsaicin and oleoresins which are thought to be the active constituents.

DOSAGE
TINCTURE: 5 or more drops. CAUTION – it is EXTREMELY HOT. In an emergency situation, you can actually use droppersful.

POWDER: A small pinch added to drinks or food, CAUTION – it is EXTREMELY HOT. CAUTION – start with only a small amount! Do not encapsulate. This can be too shocking to the stomach and digestion. Put a small amount in a little juice, stir and chug. Work your way up in dosage slowly. 1/8 to 1/4 teaspoon two to four times daily.

WARNING: *This product contains extremely HOT Cayenne pepper. Wash hands two or three times after handling this product. Do not touch sensitive areas of the body after handling this powder. When we mix this Capsicum powder, even some of our employees who are used to consuming hot peppers have to wear special anti-contamination suits with special forces gas masks I bought in Germany. I am not joking.*

For price and quantity information please refer to your American Botanical Pharmacy 2001 Herbal Product Catalog or call 1-800-HERBDOC for your FREE copy.

DR. SCHULZE'S D-TOX FORMULA

BOTANICAL INGREDIENTS *Red Clover blossoms, Trifolium pratense,* **Mojave Chaparral herb & resin,** *Larrea californica,* **Oregon Grape root,** *Berberis aquifolium,* **Burdock root & seed,** *Arctium lappa,* **Yellow Dock root,** *Rumex crispus,* **Goldenseal root,** *Hydrastis canadensis,* **Garlic juice,** *Allium sativum,* **Cayenne peppers,** *Capsicum annum,* **Poke root,** *Phytolacca Bloodroot,* **and Lobelia seeds,** *Lobelia inflata.*

METABOLIC ACTION AND BOTANICAL CHEMISTRY The following is common knowledge from highly respected and accepted medical texts. According to pharmacology manuals, Chaparral contains Nordihydroguaiaretic acid. According to the Merck Index, one of the most respected medical chemical books in the world, this acid from chaparral is listed as an anti-oxidant with a Therapeutic Category as an Anti-neoplastic. According to Taber's Cyclopedic Medical Dictionary, an Anti-neoplastic is "an agent that prevents the development, growth and proliferation of malignant cells."

DOSAGE
The herbs in this formula are extremely strong in taste. Dilute in a few ounces of fresh juice; grape works the best.
For general use: 2 droppersful (60 drops) 3 to 4 times a day for a week. You must consume the entire bottle during the 5 Day Cleansing Program or as described in the Incurables Program. Drink 64-128 ounces of liquid a day while taking this formula.

For price and quantity information please refer to your American Botanical Pharmacy 2001 Herbal Product Catalog or call 1-800-HERBDOC for your FREE copy.

> **"Getting well is EASY! Just STOP what you did that made you sick and START new programs that will make you healthy."**
> **- Dr. Richard Schulze**

CHAPTER 6

IMMUNOLOGY, CANCER AND AIDS

IMMUNOLOGY

Your immune system is a unique system of your body meaning it is comprised of many different types of organs, tissues, cells and fluids located throughout your body. The major components are cells, a lymphatic system including vessels, ducts and nodes, bone marrow, lymphoid aggregations like the tonsils, adenoids, Peyer's patches and appendix, the thymus, and the spleen.

This system has one main objective – to protect you from harmful alien invaders or self-mutating invaders. These invaders are often referred to as antigens (anti-creation or life) or pathogens (disease-creation). These harmful microorganisms include bacteria, virus, fungus, pollen, cancer cells, dead or old cells, and almost any substance that is not you, not self or worn out parts of you. If it is not you, or worn out, it is killed. It is that simple.

Your Immune system has two major jobs – surveillance and action. It constantly checks your blood and body for any invaders and if it detects any it goes into action.

The surveillance is achieved by the constant checking of your digestive tract, lungs, blood, virtually every cell of your body. Almost all parts of your immune system have the ability to monitor and kill.

The action it takes to destroy, neutralize and eliminate invading microrganisms is fascinating, complex, and to be honest we are far from knowing it all. There are many immune cells.

Macrophages are the big eaters, the largest of your immune cells. They eat everything in sight that isn't you. They are the garbage collectors.

T-cells – there are many different kinds with new ones being discovered occasionally. T-helper cells detect invaders and communicate enemy identification and strength while T-killer cells kill on sight and T-suppressor cells slow down the battle when it's won.

B-cells, using their surface chemical immunoglobulin, create specific poisons to kill specific invaders.

CANCER

Cancer is the second leading cause of death in the United States. Approximately 3 out of 10 people living today has or will develop cancer in their lifetime. With standard medical treatment, only forty percent of those who have cancer will survive for at least five years after their diagnosis. The most frequent sites for cancer in men are (in decreasing order) lung, colon and rectum, and prostate. In women the most frequent sites are breast, lung, colon and rectum.

Oncology is the study of neoplastic diseases. Neoplasms are made up of cells that have been changed so that their growth is excessive. These changed cells do not respond to the body's normal mechanisms for controlling cell growth. Normal cells stop growing according to a program in your genetic material (your DNA). The DNA of the cell has the time of the cell's death programmed; it is predetermined. This is called programmed cell death, and it is a normal process. To avoid overcrowding, they also stop growing if they are touching too many other cells around them. This is a feedback mechanism that stops the cells from growing too much and keeps them in balance. So, what does it mean if you have cells that don't stop growing? The regular cells in our bodies are constantly dying and being replaced by new cells. In this way, our bodies and organs remain the same size. Old, worn-out cells are replaced by new cells. Cancer cells are always being produced, but they do not ever die. They do not follow the program. They don't stop growing if they run into other cells around them, even if that means that the cells are overcrowded. This is why tumors grow bigger.

Neoplasms are classified into two categories – malignant and benign. <u>Malignant</u> neoplasms invade surrounding tissues and spread to other parts of the body. When a neoplasm spreads to a different part of the body, it is called a metastasis. The process of spreading is called metastasizing. In contrast to malignant neoplasms, <u>benign</u> neoplasms do not invade tissues nor metastasize. It's usually a relief when the doctor says the tumor is benign because we know a benign tumor does not spread to other parts of the body.

<u>GLOSSARY OF IMMUNOLOGY TERMINOLOGY</u>

Autoimmune disease	a disease in which the body's immune system attacks itself. Sometimes particular organs and tissues are involved. Examples are lupus, rheumatoid arthritis, pernicious anemia, Hashimoto's thyroiditis, Myasthenia Gravis, Graves' disease, hemolytic anemia, etc.
Carcinogenic	causes cancer
Carcinogen	substance that is known to cause cancer
Carcinoma	new growth or malignant tumor that occurs in epithelial tissue. Epithelial tissue is composed of cells that form the outer surface of the body and line the body cavities and the principal tubes and passageways leading to the exterior.
Carcinosarcoma	having characteristics of both a carcinoma and a sarcoma
Cd4	HIV attaches itself to this protein on the surface of the cell to attack white blood cells.

Dysplasia   abnormal development of tissue; abnormal changes in the tissue as a protection mechanism against a long-term source of chronic irritation

Lymph nodes   collection of lymph tissue found at intervals along the course of the lymph vessels throughout the body. The white blood cells contained in the node begin the process of inflammation and the immune attack against foreign substances.

Lymphocyte   type of white blood cell. Subtypes: helper, suppressor, natural killer, etc.

Macrophages   white blood cells located in all the tissues of the body that attack and digest foreign material by phagocytosis. Example: Kupffer cells in the liver

Monocyte   type of white blood cell

Neutrophil   type of white blood cell

Lupus   Systemic Lupus Erythematosus (SLE for short)

Lymphoma   cancer of the lymph nodes

Metaplasia   (from meta - meaning change or transformation, and plassein – to form) conversion of one kind of tissue into a form that is not normal for that tissue. For example, in a condition called Barrett's esophagus, some esophagus cells are converted to stomach cells. The stomach cells are normal, but they do not belong in the esophagus. Usually, there is some sort of irritation that causes this process to happen. For example, when the acid washes up out of the stomach into the esophagus, those cells have to change into stomach cells because stomach cells have characteristics that protect them from stomach acid. This is a protective mechanism. (See how your body is always trying to protect itself and survive?) Chronic metaplasia (metaplasia that exists in the body for a long period of time) can eventually lead to dysplasia.

Metastasis   movement of cancer cells from one part of the body to another. The malignant cells may spread through the lymphatic circulation, the bloodstream, or other ways such as through the cerebrospinal fluid.

Phagocyte   cell that ingests and digests bacteria and other particles through the process of phagocytosis

Red blood cells   cells in the blood that give it its characteristic red color. Red blood cells contain hemoglobin which carry oxygen.

Sarcoma   cancer arising from connective tissue such as muscle or bone, which may affect the bones, bladder, kidneys, liver, lungs, parotids, and spleen

Staging   process of determining how big a malignant tumor is and how much it has spread or not spread. Staging usually determines chances for recovery and survival. Cancer is classified into different stages according to the type of cancer. e.g. colon cancer – Duke stages

Tumor markers   substances found in the blood that indicate the presence of cancer. Examples are CA-125: ovarian cancer and others, CEA : embryonic antigen – digestive cancers, and PSA : prostate specific antigen (only if the level is above 4) indicates prostate cancer.

White blood cells cells in the blood that make up the immune system

SPECIFIC HERBAL FORMULAE FOR THE IMMUNE SYSTEM

DR. SCHULZE'S ECHINACEA PLUS

BOTANICAL INGREDIENTS *Wild-harvested Echinacea fresh root and juice,* *Echinacea angustifolia,* **Organic Echinacea seed,** *Echinacea purpurea,* **Organic Garlic juice,** *Allium sativum,* **and Organic Habanero Cayenne pepper and juice,** *Capsicum annum.*

METABOLIC ACTION In the past decade, hundreds of medical and scientific articles have been written exalting Echinacea's immune stimulating competency and scientifically explaining how it works.

Simply put, **Echinacea** works in two main ways. First, it builds up your immune system by stimulating you to build more immune cells and immune chemicals. Secondly, it also stimulates these immune cells into action and heightened activity levels. These actions will help you combat any infection or disease more effectively and also protect you from future invasion and illness.

Echinacea is one of the strongest immune stimulators and enhancers known. It can double and triple the amount of T-cells and Macrophages in your bloodstream and increase the number of Granulocytes. It also stimulates the phagocytosis, the ability to kill and eat the bad guys, in all of these white blood cells. Echinacea can also increase the amount of Interferon, Interleukin, Immunoglobulin and other important natural immune chemicals present in your blood. Again, **this is how Echinacea works, by boosting the number of immune cells and the amount of natural immune chemicals in your body and then stimulating them into being more active.** This is why in my clinic, Echinacea Plus was an extremely effective treatment, not only for acute infections, but also for long term diseases.

There are literally hundreds of other known and researched healing and protecting abilities of Echinacea besides colds, flu, sore throats and upper respiratory infections. A partial list includes inhibiting tumor growth, killing strep and staph bacteria, halting urinary tract infections, healing infected wounds, relieving hives and allergic reactions, stopping allergies, neutralizing toxic and poisonous insect and animal bites and stings, etc.

Echinacea Plus also contains **Garlic**, one of the strongest medicinal plants on earth. It is a supreme infection fighter capable of killing all bacteria, virus and fungus on contact. Unlike Echinacea, that can only be documented in Native American Indian usage back to the 17th century, the medicinal use of Garlic has been documented, if not worshiped since the beginning of recorded history. From the Egyptians and Greeks to the Romans, Garlic was used as both food and strong medicine to strengthen and heal the body. In research it has been diluted 1 part in 125,000 and still killed bacteria. In fact, just the odor has proven to be highly antibacterial. It is an extremely effective and powerful broad-spectrum antibiotic, which means it kills all types of bacteria on contact, gram positive and gram negative. Garlic's use as an anti-bacterial drug in Russia is so esteemed it has been nicknamed Russian penicillin. Garlic has been proven to destroy many types of bacteria including Streptococcus, Staphylococcus, Typhoid, Diphtheria, Cholera, E. coli, Bacterial Dysentery (Travelers' diarrhea), Tuberculosis, Tetanus, Rheumatic bacteria and many others.

Garlic is also a very powerful anti-viral agent proven in the laboratory. Many doctors feel it's the cure for the common cold. It destroys various viruses that cause upper respiratory infections and influenza, the ones that antibiotics are useless against. Garlic destroys on contact the viral infections of Measles, Mumps, Mononucleosis, Chicken pox, Herpes simplex #1 and #2, Herpes zoster, Viral Hepatitis, Scarlet fever, Rabies and others. So while some say that the reason you don't catch colds when you eat garlic is because no one will come near you, remember that garlic is also a powerful anti-viral agent. Some people ask: Why do I use Garlic instead of Goldenseal root? There is really no contest. Goldenseal is a mild anti-bacterial bitter herb. It is wonderful for the sensitive areas of the body and sinus complaints, but compared to Garlic, GET REAL! Echinacea and Garlic, not the fad-ish goldenseal, are the *Herbal Dynamic Duo*. Echinacea will enhance, stimulate and strengthen your immune system to protect you, and Garlic will destroy the invader on sight.

Habanero pepper, which is unique to my formula, increases your blood and lymph circulation which makes this formula ten times more effective than Echinacea by itself.

BOTANICAL CHEMISTRY Echinacea contains phytochemicals such as Polysaccharides, Isobutyl amides, Polyacetylenes, Cichoric Acid, Echinacoside and Cynarin. These chemicals are known to produce many healing benefits such as

Hyaluronidase inhibition which protects your cells by stopping bacteria, viruses and other disease causing organisms from being able to penetrate your cellular walls. These chemicals also stimulate and increase the number of leukocytes (white blood cells) in your body. These cells, T-cells, B-cells, Granualocytes, Macrophages, etc, are some of the main components of your immune system that directly kill and eat bacteria and viruses. These and other chemicals in Echinacea increase phagocytosis, the ability and speed of the above mentioned cells to destroy and dispose of bacteria, viruses, fungi and other disease causing microbes. Echinacea increases production of gamma globulins. These are the chemicals that coat your B-cells which are used to make antibodies. Antibodies are chemicals that kill specific bacteria, viruses and other pathogens that can hurt you and make you sick.

Garlic contains over 80 different sulfur compounds which make it such a powerful infection fighter. It also contains allicin, which is one of the strongest disease and infection fighters found in Nature.

DOSAGE

The dosage is dependent on the situation. My suggested clinical dosages are as follows, which I might mention are double what most other armchair herbalists suggest. But these dosages created successful healings in my clinic year after year. Oddly enough, the most effective dosage and treatment using Echinacea is like a treatment of antibiotics. Echinacea must be taken steadily over a period of about 2 weeks for maximum immune protection.

FOR PREVENTATIVE IMMUNE BOOSTING, BUT WITH NO CURRENT HEALTH PROBLEM:

For general protection and immune stimulation, especially when you are not ill. This could be even when you're feeling fine, but many around you are ill. People asked me for years, "How can you be around so many sick people all the time and stay healthy yourself?" Well, I live a very healthy lifestyle and take lots of Echinacea Plus.

Use 2 droppersful (about 60 drops), five times daily until you have consumed 2 fluid ounces or 60 milliliters. This will take about seven days. Do this at the beginning of each month in the Winter season for the best cold and flu prevention.

YOU HAVE THAT UH-OH FEELING, NO SPECIFIC SYMPTOMS BUT YOU THINK YOU'RE "COMING DOWN WITH SOMETHING":

When you're feeling out of sorts or a bit off, but it's nothing you can really put your finger on, this may mean that you are about to get sick. It also may mean that your body is fighting something off. But in either case it is a good time to give it some help. **In this scenario use 4 droppersful (about 120 drops) five times daily until you have consumed 2 fluid ounces or 60 milliliters.** This will take about three to four days.

ONSET OF FEVER, CHILLS OR ANY OF THE SYMPTOMS OF A COLD OR FLU:

This is when you actually have some observable, clinical symptoms: sore throat, fever, nasal or lung congestion, toxic bite or sting, wound or trauma. Anytime there is anything wrong with you, your immune system must go to work.

Use 4 droppersful (about 120 drops), eight times daily (or every other hour you are awake) until you have consumed 2 fluid ounces or 60 milliliters. This will take about two days. You may continue this dosage for a week and then reduce dosage.

HIGH FEVER, SORE THROAT, YELLOW MUCOUS, COUGHING, SNEEZING:

This is when you are suddenly sweating, have the chills, a cold, food poisoning or any serious illness: you are really ill. There is no time to waste fooling around; immediate aggressive herbal treatment is indicated. **In this case use 1 fluid ounce of Echinacea Plus immediately. For those who might have a hard time doing this, it can be diluted in juice or drunk 1/2 ounce one hour and the other 1/2 ounce the next.** Remember that this is one ounce of alcohol so keep that in mind and don't drive. Then consume an additional ounce during the rest of the day. The following days consume at least one, if not two fluid ounces of Echinacea Plus every day until you feel the infection break.

REMEMBER, all of the above suggested dosages can be doubled, tripled, even quadrupled; meaning you can consume more than 2 fluid ounces a day if desired. Many of my patients doubled, tripled, even quadrupled these suggestions. It is important to note that there are no toxic side effects with Echinacea and no known overdoses. Health circle rumors abound that if you take too much Echinacea or take it for too long you could **"burn out your immune system."** Over the years in my clinic, I had many an Echinacea **junkie** and never saw one case of a depressed immunity because of their habit and subsequent overdoses. I had many patients who took Echinacea every day for two to three years without a break. All I saw were miracle healings. On the contrary, I saw many people stay sick and not recover because they didn't take enough herbs.

Echinacea is a strong medicinal herb. All medicinal and toning herbs are best used for a period of time and then stopped for a week or two. This is true of most medicinal herbs.

For price and quantity information please refer to your American Botanical Pharmacy 2001 Herbal Product Catalog or call 1-800-HERBDOC for your FREE copy.

DR. SCHULZE'S LIVER/GALLBLADDER & ANTI-PARASITE FORMULA

BOTANICAL INGREDIENTS *Milk Thistle seed,* Silybum marianum, **Dandelion root,** *Taraxacum officinale,* **Oregon Grape root,** *Berberis aquifolium,* **Gentian root,** *Gentiana lutea,* **Wormwood leaf and flower,** *Artemisia Absinthium,* **Mojave Chaparral herb,** *Larrea californica,* **Black Walnut hulls,** *Juglans nigra,* **Ginger rhizome,** *Zingiber officinale,* **Garlic bulb,** *Allium sativum,* **and Fennel seed,** *Foeniculum officinale.*

METABOLIC ACTION AND BOTANICAL CHEMISTRY The herbs in this formula are famous for their ability to stimulate, cleanse and protect the liver and gallbladder and rid the body of parasites. **Milk Thistle** contains many phytochemicals, three chief ones being silibinin, silydianin and silychristin. These three plant chemicals are often collectively referred to as *silymarin*. There are many ways in which these plant chemicals protect and heal your liver, too many for this book. But two main ones are **protection** and **regeneration**. **The phytochemicals in Milk Thistle actually strengthen the structure of the hepatocytes (liver cells) skin or membrane which prevents the penetration of known liver toxins.**

These protective chemicals also stimulate the action of the nucleolar polymerase A, resulting in an increase in ribosomal protein synthesis and thus stimulate the regeneration of damaged liver cells and stimulate the formation of new liver cells. These chemicals are so powerful they can even protect you from some of the most lethal poisons on the planet, like death-cap mushrooms. Simply put, ingesting Milk thistle is like putting a protective coating around your current liver cells while it speeds repair of damaged ones and builds new strong cells.

Oregon Grape rootbark, Gentian root, Wormwood leaves and **Dandelion root** are some of the most bitter plants on the planet and all classic bitter liver tonic herbs. They contain phytochemicals like berberine alkaloids and volatile oils which stimulate the liver to produce more bile which will flush out the bile ducts and gallbladder.

The **Black Walnut hulls, Wormwood** and **Garlic** are strong ANTI-PARASITICAL plants. Parasite infestation is a fact of life. One cubic inch of choice beef can have over 1,000 living parasite larvae waiting to hatch in your body. Over 65% of fresh fish tested had toxic levels of bacteria and parasites. Chicken is even worse. I've had hundreds of patients expel toilet bowls full of intestinal parasites, including tape worms over 30 FEET LONG. They have also killed cellular parasites with this formula. It works best if used in conjunction with both Intestinal Formulas #1 and #2. Use if parasites are suspected, or if there has been a history of bowel problems, constipation, eating of animal products, prolonged illness, disease and degeneration. If you have been exposed to any toxic substances, or drank alcohol or other harmful beverages, this formula is for you. It is also beneficial if you have had high cholesterol, blood fats or any family history of liver or gallbladder problems. Many believe that anyone who has cancer or any immune dysfunction had a weak congested liver to begin with. Even if a person had their gallbladder removed, these herbs will still be effective in cleaning the liver and bile ducts.

DOSAGE

2 droppersful (60 drops) three to four times daily for 1 week. This formula is most effective if used in conjunction with the Detoxification Tea and also my 5 Day Cleansing and Detoxification Program with the Liver/Gallbladder Flush.

For price and quantity information please refer to your American Botanical Pharmacy 2001 Herbal Product Catalog or call 1-800-HERBDOC for your FREE copy.

CHAPTER 7

MALE AND FEMALE REPRODUCTIVE SYSTEMS

EXPLANATION OF SYSTEM

THE MALE REPRODUCTIVE SYSTEM

The male reproductive organs produce spermatozoa, the male reproductive cells, and are used for sexual intercourse. They are made up of internal and external organs. The internal organs include the testes (testicles), epididymis, vas deferens, seminal vesicles, ejaculatory ducts, and the prostate gland. The external organs include the penis and scrotum.

The average length of the penis at rest is about eight centimeters. It consists of a cylinder-shaped shaft and the glans at the tip. The urethra passes through the length of the penis and opens to the outside of the body at the end of the glans. The shaft of the penis is formed by the corpus cavernosum in the back and a spongy structure called the corpus spongiosum toward the end. These structures are meshlike and contain lots of empty spaces. When blood from the branches of the central artery of the penis fills these spaces (venous cavities), the penis swells. This is how an erection occurs.

The testis is approximately 4-5 centimeters in length and is shaped somewhat like a flat egg. Each testis lies inside each scrotum. Rolled up within each testis are approximately 1000 seminiferous tubules, each of which is almost one meter in length when stretched out. These tubules begin to produce spermatozoa at puberty. The tubules straighten out at

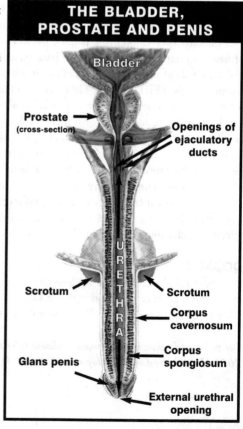

THE BLADDER, PROSTATE AND PENIS

Bladder

Prostate (cross-section) →

Openings of ejaculatory ducts

Scrotum

Scrotum

Corpus cavernosum

Corpus spongiosum

Glans penis

External urethral opening

URETHRA

the end of the scrotum, and these straight tubules then carry the spermatozoa to the epididymis. The interstitial tissue filling the space between the seminiferous tubules contains interstitial cells that secrete the male hormone testosterone.

The epididymis is a twisted mass of long ducts, each of which is as long as six meters when stretched out. The spermatozoa from the testis are stored here for ten to twenty days. The spermatozoa are then carried in tubules to the seminal vesicles which are two sacs that lie on either side of the prostate gland. The seminal vesicles produce a fluid called semen in which the spermatozoa can "swim". The semen then goes to the prostate gland which also produces additional fluid for the sperm. The semen goes to the urethra where it will be carried through the penis to the outside of the body. The urethra is the tubule that also carries urine from the bladder through the penis to the outside of the body.

The prostate gland surrounds the urethra, so when the prostate enlarges due to benign prostatic hypertrophy (BPH), it narrows the urethra which carries the urine to the outside. Eventually, the urine flow is slowed and blocked so much that it can back up into the kidneys and cause kidney damage.

THE FEMALE REPRODUCTIVE SYSTEM

The female reproductive organs are responsible for the production of eggs, (the female reproductive cells) and after fertilization, they are involved in the development and birth of the fetus. The internal organs are the ovaries, uterus, fallopian tubes and the vagina. The external organs are the labia minora and majora, the clitoris and the vestibule of the vagina.

The ovaries are shaped like ovals. They are located on the left and right side of the uterus just below the two fallopian tubes. The ovaries are approximately 2.5 to 4 centimeters in length, 1.2 to 2 centimeters in width and approximately 1 centimeter thick. They produce microscopic eggs called ova one of which, when combined with a spermatozoa during fertilization, grows into a fetus. The ovaries also produce a variety of hormones.

Inside the cortex layer of each ovary are a certain number of immature eggs called ova which are contained in follicles. The ova are in various stages of maturing. Follicle stimulating hormones (FSH) causes the follicles to mature, and luteinizing hormones (LH) cause the mature follicle to break open and release the ova. This process is known as ovulation. This is the time when a woman is considered "fertile" – when she can get pregnant. Normally, one egg is released alternately each month either from the left or the right ovary. About 500 eggs are released in a lifetime. The follicles that remain after release of the ovum become corpus luteum which secretes progesterone. The ovum then enters the fallopian tube on that side, and if it is not fertilized by a sperm, it dies and is reabsorbed by the body. If the ovum is fertilized and pregnancy occurs, the progesterone produced by the corpus luteum provides hormonal support for the pregnancy. If fertilization does not occur, the corpus luteum degenerates.

If the fallopian tube is scarred (usually from a sexually transmitted disease that causes an infection of the fallopian tubes, called Pelvic Inflammatory Disease or PID), the egg does not make it to the uterus and can still be fertilized in the tube. This causes a tubal pregnancy, also called an ectopic pregnancy, which becomes a life-threatening situation when the fetus grows and bursts the tube.

The uterus is a muscular, hollow, pear-shaped structure which leans forward over and just behind the bladder. It also lies in front of the colon. The uterus consists of the body, the isthmus and the cervix. The cervix is the lowermost cylinder-shaped portion that joins the uterus to the upper end of the vagina.

The inner surface of the uterus is lined by a mucous membrane called the endometrium. The endometrium peels away during menstruation. The normal menstrual cycle (from the first day of one menstrual period to the first day of the next) is about 25-28 days. The normal level of menstrual blood flow varies from 20-120 milliliters. Ovulation usually occurs in the middle of the menstrual cycle, or around day fourteen.

If fertilization occurs, the fertilized ovum will implant in the endometrium which will begin to grow and develop under the influence of hormones secreted by the ovary (progesterone and estrogen). About five weeks later, the fertilized ovum and the endometrium will form the placenta which supplies the growing fetus with blood and nourishment. The normal uterus is around seven centimeters long. It can expand during pregnancy to about 36 centimeters in length. In just over nine months, the space within the uterus enlarges 2000-2500 times.

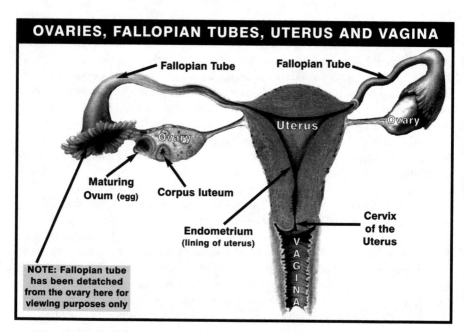

OVARIES, FALLOPIAN TUBES, UTERUS AND VAGINA

GLOSSARY OF MALE AND FEMALE REPRODUCTIVE SYSTEM TERMINOLOGY

Amenorrhea   absence of flow and menstruation, normal before puberty and after menopause

Cervix   the part of any organ that resembles the neck, in this case the uterus

Corpus Luteum   small yellow body that develops within a ruptured ovarian follicle; endocrine structure that secretes progesterone

D and C   *dilation* of the cervix and *curettage* of the uterus, a surgical procedure that involves scraping of the inside of the uterus; used therapeutically for excessive vaginal bleeding or to abort a fetus

Dysmenorrhea   dys = abnormal, bad, difficult, painful   men = month   rhea = to flow painful or difficult menstruation

Dysplasia   abnormal development of tissue

Dyspareunia   pain in the labia, uterus or vagina during or after sex; an abnormal occurrence which usually indicates disease, infection or some other condition

Endometriosis   ectopic endometrium located in various sites throughout the pelvis or abdominal wall

Endometritis   inflammation of endometrium, usually bacterial, staphylococci, E. coli bacilli, gonococci, or trauma

Endometrium   mucous membrane lining the inner surface of the uterus

Endocrine Gland   gland that secretes directly into the bloodstream

Estrogen   (Greek = oistroos / mad desire + gennan / to produce, the Estrogenic hormones Estradiol and Estrone (together they produce Estriol) produced by the ovary; the female sex hormones which create cyclic changes in the uterus (menstruation)

Fallopian Tube   tube/duct that extends from the end of the uterus and terminates near the ovary

Fertilization	union of an ovum and a spermatazoon, usually taking place in the fallopian tube
Fibroids	benign encapsulated tumors of the uterus; they usually result in pain and excess bleeding
FSH	Follicle Stimulating Hormone, produced by the anterior pituitary; stimulates growth of the follicle in the ovary and spermatogenesis in the testis
Gonad	generic term for an ovary or testicle
Gonadotrophic Hormones	see Gonadotropin
Gonadotropin	gonad stimulating hormone; stimulates the ovaries and testes
Gonadotropin Releasing Hormone	produced in the hypothalamus, acts on the pituitary to cause the release of the Gonadotrophic Hormones FSH, LH and ICSH
Hormone	(Greek, hormon = urging on) a substance originating in an organ or gland which is conveyed through the bloodstream to another part of the body; stimulating it by chemical action to increase functional activity or to increase the secretion of another hormone
Hypothalamus	A part of the brain that lies beneath the thalamus. It contains neurosecretions that control many metabolic activities from water balance to sugar and fat metabolism; regulates body temperature and secretes releasing and inhibiting hormones
Hysterectomy	surgical removal of the uterus; often combined with a salpingo-oophorectomy – removal of the fallopian tubes and ovaries
LH	Luteinizing Hormone which stimulates development of the Corpus Luteum
Menopause	period which marks the permanent cessation of menstrual activity

Menstruation	periodic discharge of bloody fluid from the uterus at intervals between puberty and menopause. The discharge contains blood, disintegrated endometrial cells and secretions of glands. This blood does not coagulate but does include clots. Menstruation is brought on by the reduction in production of ovarian hormones, especially progesterone. This results in involution of the Corpus Luteum following failure of the ovum to become fertilized.
Ovary	one of two glands in the female that produces the reproductive cell, the ovum. The ovary also produces two known hormones – estrogen, which is secreted by the follicles and progesterone, which is secreted by the corpus luteum
Ovum	female reproductive cell
Pap Smear/Test	Papanicolaou test used supposedly for early detection of cancer cells
Pituitary Gland	small endocrine gland attached to the base of the brain which secretes a number of different hormones that regulate many bodily functions such as growth and reproduction; often referred to as the master gland
Polycystic ovarian disease	the presence of many cysts in the ovaries which usually leads to pain and infertility
Progesterone	steroid hormone responsible for changes in the uterine endometrium in the second half of the menstrual cycle; used to treat menstrual disorders and threatened abortion
Prostate	gland that surrounds the neck of the bladder and urethra in the male, part muscle and part gland; has ducts that open into the urethra; produces some of the seminal fluid
Prostatitis	inflammation of the prostate
Puberty	period of life when either sex becomes functionally capable of reproduction; usually occuring between the ages of 9 to 16 in girls and 13 to 15 in boys and ends in the attainment of sexual maturity
Sperm	ejaculate of the male
Spermatozoa	mature male sex cell formed in the testis

Steroid   large group of chemicals related to sterols; some hormones fall into this category

Testicle   a testis, one of two reproductive glands located in the scrotum that produce the male reproductive cells, the spermatozoa, and the male hormone testosterone

Testosterone   principal testicular hormone produced in men. It accelerates the growth of tissue and stimulates blood flow. It stimulates and promotes the growth of sexual characteristics and is essential for normal sexual behavior.

SPECIFIC HERBAL FORMULAE FOR THE MALE AND FEMALE REPRODUCTIVE SYSTEMS

DR. SCHULZE'S FEMALE FORMULA

BOTANICAL INGREDIENTS *Dong Quai*, Angelica polymorpha sinensis root, *Chaste Tree berry*, Vitex agnus-castus, *Wild Yam*, Dioscorea villosa root, *Damiana leaf*, Turnera aphrodisiaca, *Licorice root*, Glycyrrhiza glabra *and Hops flowers*, Humulus lupulus.

METABOLIC ACTION AND BOTANICAL CHEMISTRY I used this herbal formula in my clinic with tremendous success. It regulates and balances female hormones during puberty, PMS and menopause and alleviates symptoms such as menstrual cramps, headaches, sensitive breasts, mood swings, anxiety, insomnia, irritability, depression, anger, nervousness, water retention/bloating, weight gain, hot flashes, hair loss and dry vaginal tissue.

It regulates and normalizes the menstrual cycle and relieves associated menstrual problems. It increases fertility and sexual desire and calms the nerves. **It is a powerfully effective overall female tonic.**

Dong Quai, Chaste Tree and **Wild Yam** are the three most popular herbs for female complaints in Traditional Chinese, European and American Herbal Medicine respectively.

It is estimated that over one billion women worldwide have used **Dong Quai** and praise this plant as a lifesaver for hormonal imbalance. For many years it has been the #1 herb sold in the world. Regardless of this massive use and clinical success, American medical doctors smugly say that there is no scientific data to back up this empirical clinical finding. I know doctors are often stupid, but to argue with a billion women?

On the other hand, **Chaste Tree berry** has had a tremendous amount of clinical findings, and scientific research is proving its effectiveness. It is documented in clinical trials to balance female hormones and successfully treat everything from acne, menstrual problems and PMS (an 86% success rate), to poor lactation and fibroid tumors.

Wild Yam root actually contains plant sources of steroids. At one time, this herb was the sole source of chemicals used in manufacturing hormones, before medicine decided horse piss was better. Cheaper is more like it! This valuable herb has been successfully and clinically proven to help with a myriad of female hormone imbalance problems.

All of the chemicals in these three powerful herbs are thought to affect the Pituitary and Hypothalmus in the brain, which both control the manufacture and release of hormones from the ovaries through the release of metabolic chemicals like gonodatropin releasing hormone.

Damiana leaf may have been one of the most widely used herbs in all of history in times gone by. It is like the female version of what Ginseng is to a man, a powerful strengthener and aphrodisiac (sexual stimulant).

Both **Licorice root** and **Hops flowers** contain phytosterols, chemical precursors to hormones. Throughout history these herbs have been used to treat hormone imbalance and just about every female problem known. They not only give women that sense of well-being and control, but allow women to age slowly and naturally and make comfortable transitions from puberty through menopause and beyond. These herbs are literally blessings from God.

DOSAGE

Dosage for Menopause: Start with 1 dropperful (30 drops) three times daily for at least one week. If this is not enough and symptoms still persist, increase to 1 dropperful four times daily. If needed, you can increase to 6 droppersful daily, but spread them out.

If your symptoms intensify during a particular time of the day or evening, use more of the formula during that time. For example, for nighttime sweats, take 2 to 3 droppersful before bedtime to offset this situation.

Dosage for PMS: For a regular 28 day cycle, on the 18th day after the start of your last period, take 1 dropperful in the morning and 1 in the evening. On the 20th day through the start of your next period, take 1 dropperful three times daily. This dosage can be increased to 2 droppersful three times daily with an occasional dosage of up to 4 droppersful during extreme symptoms. Discontinue the formula once your period begins unless you have extreme menstrual problems.

Dosage for Menstrual Irregularity: If you have had long term menstrual irregularity, start by taking 1 dropperful three times daily for 1 to 2 months. This should balance your hormones and regulate your periods.

If it is for menstrual problems during your period, take 1 to 3 droppersful three times daily as needed.

Dosage for Infertility: Start with 1 dropperful three times daily for a month. The next month you can increase to 2 droppersful three times daily. Continue with the formula. Stop if you become pregnant. As with most situations, but especially with infertility, you must do all of the foundational programs to get the best results.

For price and quantity information please refer to your American Botanical Pharmacy 2001 Herbal Product Catalog or call 1-800-HERBDOC for your FREE copy.

DR. SCHULZE'S FEMALE BALANCE

BOTANICAL INGREDIENTS *Dong Quai, Angelica polymorpha sinensis root,* **Chaste Tree,** *Vitex agnus-castus berry,* **Wild Yam,** *Dioscorea villosa root,* **Valerian root,** *Valeriana officinalis,* **Lobelia pod and seed,** *Lobelia inflata,* **Passion flower,** *Passiflora incarnata,* **Hops flower,** *Humulus lupulus,* **Uva Ursi leaf,** *Arctostaphlos uva ursi,* **Juniper berries,** *Juniperus communis* **and Corn Silk,** *Zea mays.*

METABOLIC ACTION AND BOTANICAL CHEMISTRY The nervine and antispasmodic herbs added in this formula are for treating the common PMS symptoms of sensitive breasts, mood swings, anxiety, anger, irritability, insomnia, depression and general nervousness. Another very common complaint of PMS is excess weight gain and bloating due to fluid and water retention. This is why I also added the diuretic herbs to relieve these symptoms. **Dong Quai, Chaste Tree, Wild Yam** (see Female Formula, previous page), **Valerian root, Lobelia pod** and **seed, Passion flower, Hops flower** (see Nerve and Lobelia, chapter 8), **Uva Ursi leaf, Juniper berries, Corn Silk** (see Kidney/Bladder Formula, chapter 4.)

DOSAGE

For general use take 2 droppersful three to four times daily. Up to 8 droppersful can be taken at once for PMS emergencies.

Dosage for PMS: For a regular 28 day cycle, on the 18th day after the start of your last period, take 1 dropperful in the morning and 1 in the evening. On the 20th day through the start of your next period take 1 dropperful three times daily. This dosage can be increased to 2 droppersful three times daily with an occasional dosage of up to 4 droppersful during extreme symptoms. Discontinue the formula once your period begins unless you have extreme menstrual problems.

PMS Lifestyle Modification: During PMS, what I call behavior and lifestyle modification is of great importance. Don't set yourself up for failure. If you know that for the last seven days before your next period you have bad PMS, until it is under control, again, DON'T SET YOURSELF UP FOR FAILURE! What I mean is first, don't go clothes shopping, especially with friends. Everything will be tight because of your water retention and you will hate yourself. I have had hundreds of crying women come into my clinic describing themselves as looking like a whale. Don't do this to yourself. Also do not set up any meetings with your boyfriend, husband or boss that you know will be tense or intense. Meetings especially like future projects, budgets, house remodeling and definitely not where is our marriage or relationship going. Look I had thousands of women patients with severe PMS. Heed my advice. Use PMS and menstruation as a time to celebrate your womanhood with hot baths, candles, essential oils, relaxing music, meditation and some laughs. Set yourself up to win!

DR. SCHULZE'S MALE FORMULA

BOTANICAL INGREDIENTS *Wild American "Blue Ridge" Ginseng root, Panax quinquifolium,* **Chinese and Korean Ginseng roots,** *Panax ginseng,* **Siberian Ginseng root,** *Eleutherococcus senticosus,* **Saw Palmetto berry,** *Serenoa repens,* **Sarsaparilla root,** *Smilax ornate,* **Yohimbe bark,** *Corynanthe yohimbe,* **Oat seed,** *Avena sativa,* **Kola nut,** *Cola acuminata,* **and Ginger rhizome,** *Zingiber officinale.*

METABOLIC ACTION AND BOTANICAL CHEMISTRY This is male, high-octane super fuel. This is a powerful formula, it provides men with herbal phytochemicals that are documented to create hormones, help stimulate male energy, sexual desire, promote more frequent, harder erections and for longer durations. It will also increase sperm production. **Wild American "Blue Ridge" Ginseng root, Chinese and Korean Ginseng roots, and Siberian Ginseng root** (see Super Ginseng Blend) are famous all over the world, and have been for thousands of years. Medical texts report that Ginseng strengthens the body and increases its resistance to fatigue, and also increases your capacity for work and concentration. Regardless, these herbs have been prized the world over. In fact, wars have been fought over them, because men say that Ginseng effects their sexual desire and function.

Yohimbe bark, like Ginseng, is famous worldwide as a male aphrodisiac and sexual stimulant, but medicine fails to comment and only says that it increases nervous excitation. **Oat seed** and **Kola nut** both fall into this same category.

Sarsaparilla root: several species of this plant at various times in history were as popular as Ginseng. Although it contains steroidal compounds, little research has been done on this plant. **Saw Palmetto berry** (See Prostate Formula, next page). Regardless of modern medicine's lack of opinion and research on most of these plants, they are considered the most powerful male herbs on the planet and have been used for centuries for this purpose.

DOSAGE

2 droppersful (30-60 drops) three to four times daily. Works best if used consistently over a period of three to four months and of course, with all of the Foundational Programs.

For price and quantity information please refer to your American Botanical Pharmacy 2001 Herbal Product Catalog or call 1-800-HERBDOC for your FREE copy.

DR. SCHULZE'S SUPER GINSENG BLEND

BOTANICAL INGREDIENTS *Wild American Blue Ridge Ginseng, Panax quinquifolium,* **Chinese and Korean Ginseng,** *Panax ginseng,* **and Wild Siberian Ginseng,** *Eleutherococcus senticosus.*

METABOLIC ACTION AND BOTANICAL CHEMISTRY (See Male Formula on previous page.)

DOSAGE
1-2 droppersful (30-60 drops) three to four times daily. Works best if used with the **Male Formula.**

DR. SCHULZE'S PROSTATE FORMULA

BOTANICAL INGREDIENTS *Saw Palmetto berry, Serenoa repens,* **Uva Ursi leaves,** *Arctostaphlos,* **Juniper Berries,** *Juniperus communis,* **Pygeum bark,** *Pygeum africanum,* **Nettle root,** *Urtica dioica* **and Corn Silk,** *Zea mays.*

METABOLIC ACTION AND BOTANICAL CHEMISTRY Saw Palmetto, **Pygeum bark** and **Stinging Nettle root** have all been clinically established to relieve the symptoms of Benign Prostate Hypertrophy although their action is not scientifically understood. **Uva Ursi leaves, Juniper Berry** and **Corn Silk.** (See the Kidney/Bladder Formula, chapter 4.)

DOSAGE
1-2 droppersful (30-60 drops) three to four times daily. Works best if used consistently over a period of three to four months. Take an extra dropperful before bedtime if you have a problem with urinating at night. Since the consumption of all animal products, especially beef, has been directly linked as a cause of BPH, for maximum effect and disease reversal it is imperative to follow a vegetarian food program during treatment.

For price and quantity information please refer to your American Botanical Pharmacy 2001 Herbal Product Catalog or call 1-800-HERBDOC for your FREE copy.

CHAPTER 8

THE NEUROLOGICAL AND NEUROMUSCULAR SYSTEMS

EXPLANATION OF SYSTEM

The body's nervous system is divided into the central nervous system and the peripheral nervous system. The central nervous system consists of the brain and spinal cord. The brain is the site where mental activity occurs, and the brain and spinal cord together act as the center for maintaining life. The peripheral nervous system is the communication pathway connecting the central nervous system with the various parts of the body (periphery). The peripheral system is divided into the cranial nerves that lead to and from the brain and the spinal nerves that lead to and from the spinal cord. The two systems combined are also known as the cerebrospinal system.

The cranial nerves control feeling and function of the various parts of the head and face, including the muscles, eyes, ears, and nose. The spinal nerves transmit signals from the brain to the four arms and legs and the trunk and send information from the various parts of the body back to the brain and spinal cord.

The peripheral nervous system is divided into the somatic nervous system (motor and sensory nerves), which receives information from the surface of the body and controls involuntary reactions of the internal organs and blood vessels. The autonomic nervous system consists of the sympathetic and parasympathetic nervous systems that work together to maintain the internal environment of the body.

The sympathetic nervous system performs actions in the body that are referred to as the "fight or flight" mechanism. The sympathetic nervous system governs the reaction to an emergency situation: the heart rate, blood pressure, and respiratory rate increases; the pupils dilate; and the bronchioles dilate. Starches stored in the liver (glycogen) are broken down and released into the blood for quick energy – this raises the blood sugar. Also, the action of the intestinal muscles (peristalsis) slows; blood flow increases to the muscles; and the adrenal glands increase their secretion of stress hormones like cortisol, adrenaline, etc. This response prepares the body either to fight or flee.

The parasympathetic system causes the constriction of the pupil, contraction of the smooth muscles of the digestive system, narrowing of the bronchioles, slowing of the heart rate, and increased secretion by the glands, except the sweat glands. This system predominates in situations without stress. Both the sympathetic and parasympathetic nervous systems compete to keep the internal functioning of the body in balance.

Motor nerves are responsible for movement of voluntary muscles, also called skeletal muscles. Sensory nerves receive sensory information like sight, taste, touch, smell, hearing, pain, hot and cold and relay it to the brain to interpret. Voluntary muscles are under our conscious control. We decide when to move our arms, legs, etc. Involuntary muscles include the muscles of respiration, the heart, the intestinal muscles, etc. They are under the control of the autonomic nervous system. Involuntary muscles are controlled by nerves that work without our thinking about it. Involuntary muscles are also called smooth muscles. We digest food, blink, breathe, and pump blood through our bodies without our conscious control.

A single nerve cell (neuron) consists of a cell body and its projections – an axon and one or more dendrites. Neurons start and conduct nerve signals. Axons receive nerve signals from other neurons, and dendrites send signals out to other neurons. Neurons transmit signals to other neurons or cells by releasing chemicals called neurotransmitters at the gaps (synapses) between the nerves. These signals either excite or inhibit the target cells. Many axons, especially in the brain, are covered by a sheath made up of fats and lipids called myelin. Myelin acts as an electrical insulator and increases the speed of impulse transmission. Neurons can also send signals by way of releasing neurohormones into the bloodstream.

GLOSSARY OF NERVOUS SYSTEM TERMINOLOGY

A. Lateral Sclerosis   see Lou Gehrig's Disease

Alzheimer's Disease   form of dementia in which acetylcholine –transmitting neurons are affected causing the brain to shrink and fill with "plaques" and "tangles"; memory loss is the most prominent symptom

Anticonvulsants   drugs used to suppress epileptic seizures

Anxiety   vague feeling of apprehension, worry, uneasiness or dread; the source of it is often unknown to the individual

Attention Deficit Disorder   also called ADHD

Brain cancer   malignant tumor of any part of the brain – in the hemisphere, in the cerebellum, on the brain stem, etc. Patients usually have seizures, headaches, sometimes blindness, paralysis, extreme mood changes, and problems speaking.

CAT scan short for computed tomography scan; has a greater sensitivity than an x-ray since a computer takes several x-ray images and analyzes all of them together to make a 3 dimensional picture

Depression mental disorder marked by an altered mood resulting in loss of interest in all usually pleasurable outlets such as food, sex, work, friends, hobbies, or entertainment

EEG short for electroencephalogram which uses electrodes to measure the brain waves. Abnormalities of brain waves are common in brain diseases, seizures, and sleep disturbances.

EMG short for electromyography, graphic record of the contraction of a muscle which has been electrically stimulated by an instrument; test for nerve and muscle diseases

Epilepsy see seizure

Guillain-Barre Syndrome acute, usually progressive form of nerve disease characterized by muscular weakness and mild sensory loss of the extremities that often begins five days to three weeks after an infection, surgery or immunization. It begins in the legs and progresses to the arms, accompanied by a pins and needles sensation. Severe cases lead to respiratory failure, heart arrhythmias, and blood pressure abnormalities.

Lou Gehrig's Disease amyotrophic lateral sclerosis or abbreviated as A. Lateral Sclerosis or ALS; a progressive disease of the motor nerves causing muscle weakness and atrophy. Symptoms usually begin in the hand muscles accompanied by cramps and spasticity of muscles. Problems with speech and swallowing develop as a result of deterioration of nerves in the brainstem.

Lumbar Puncture also called "spinal tap". A procedure during which the doctor introduces a large needle through the back, then through the bone of the spine to reach the area of the spinal cord which is surrounded by fluid (the cerebrospinal fluid or CSF for short). Some fluid is drained from the area and is used for certain tests to determine neurologic diseases such as multiple sclerosis, infections such as meningitis, or cancers.

MRI stands for magnetic resonance imaging - a type of diagnostic radiography using electromagnetic energy. MRIs provide a clearer picture of bones, muscles, organs, and blood vessels than a CAT scan.

Multiple sclerosis	*multiple* – many, *sclerosis* – condition of hardening; a slowly progressive disease that affects several areas of the brain and spinal cord at the same time. The immune system attacks the outer covering (called the myelin sheath) of many nerves, causing various symptoms. The most common symptoms are pins and needles sensations, weakness or clumsiness of a leg or a hand, problems walking, difficulty with bladder control, emotional changes such as sudden weeping or forced laughter. Sometimes the disease affects the optic nerve resulting in partial blindness and pain in one eye, double vision, dimness of vision, or blind spots.
Muscle biopsy	surgical procedure involving cutting away a piece of muscle tissue in order to do tests to diagnose certain neuromuscular diseases.
Muscular Dystrophy	group of inherited muscle disorders of unknown cause; the most common type (Duchenne) affecting boys between the ages of 3 to 7 and causing muscle weakness of the shoulder and hip muscles. Symptoms include a waddling walk, toe-walking, spinal curvature, frequent falls, and difficulty in standing up and climbing stairs. Diagnosis is made with a muscle biopsy.
Myasthenia Gravis	an autoimmune disease marked by extreme muscle fatigue, especially with exercise. Symptoms include drooping of the upper eyelids, double vision, difficulty chewing and swallowing due to weakness of the facial muscles. It is diagnosed with the Tensilon test. Treatment is plasmapheresis and drugs that suppress the immune system.
Myelogram	x-ray of the spinal cord after injection of a contrast medium (usually a radioactive substance) into the space surrounding the spinal cord to show spinal cord tumors, herniated vertebral discs, and other abnormalities of the spine and spinal cord
Neuro	pertaining to the nerves, brain or nervous system.
Neuron	nerve cell
Optic nerve	cranial nerve responsible for vision and transmitting visual information to the brain

Parkinson's Disease   slowly progressive degenerative nervous system disorder caused by a loss of neurons in a particular area of the brain (the substantia nigra which produces a neurotransmitter called dopamine); marked by slowness of movement, muscular rigidity, a tremor at rest and an unstable posture. The characteristic "pill-rolling" tremor appears as if the patient were rolling a pill between his fingers and thumb.

Plasmapheresis   treatment for myasthenia gravis and Guillain Barre syndrome in which blood is removed from the body, and the cells and other components removed by a separator device, and the clear fluid of the blood (plasma) is returned to the body. Other substances such as immune complexes, protein-bound toxins and antibodies are also removed. It is believed that these substances contribute to the two conditions mentioned above. When removed, the patient usually experiences some relief from symptoms.

Polio   an acute viral inflammation of the gray matter of the spinal cord. The illness is usually mild lasting only a few days and affecting the respiratory and gastrointestinal systems. In the major form, muscle paralysis or weakness occurs with resulting muscle atrophy and permanent deformities.

Seizure   attack of epilepsy; a recurrent cerebral disorder marked by sudden brief attacks of altered consciousness, motor activity or sensory phenomena. Symptoms may vary from a barely noticeable lapse of consciousness to a dramatic loss of consciousness, a cry, falling, convulsions of the extremities, loss of urinary and fecal continence, and amnesia for the event. Seizures can be caused by a brain tumor, scar tissue remaining after head trauma, lack of oxygen, or sometimes there is no known cause.

Serotonin   a neurotransmitter important for the sleep-wake cycle; abnormalities in serotonin are found in depression and sleep disorders

Stroke   also called cerebrovascular accident, abbreviated as CVA. The two types are hemorrhagic stroke (bleeding in the brain usually caused by long-term high blood pressure), and ischemic stroke (cerebral blood vessels become blocked by cholesterol or a blood clot so that part of the brain dies). Symptoms include loss of consciousness, headache, loss of speech, and paralysis. Patients may or may not recover fully.

Tensilon test	diagnostic test for myasthenia gravis. An injection of Tensilon (Edrophonium) improves the symptoms of those with myasthenia gravis, thus, this test is diagnostic.
Tourette's Syndrome	nervous disorder marked by the presence of brief, rapid, involuntary muscle movements or tics. It begins with simple tics, but progresses to multiple complex movements including respiratory and vocal tics. The vocal tics may begin as grunting or barking noises and develop into compulsive utterances and often even profanity which can be physically and socially disabling. Personally I wonder why the people with Tourette's Syndrome that yell profanities never scream LOVE, BLISS, WONDERFUL, YES, etc.

SPECIFIC HERBAL FORMULAE FOR THE NERVOUS SYSTEM

DR. SCHULZE'S BRAIN FORMULA

BOTANICAL INGREDIENTS *Ginkgo Biloba leaf,* Ginkgo biloba, **Rosemary leaf and flower,** Rosmarinus officinale, **Kola nut,** Cola acuminata **and Cayenne peppers,** Capsicum annum.

METABOLIC ACTION AND BOTANICAL CHEMISTRY Recently, because of its efficacy, **Ginkgo** has become one of the most used herbs in America and the world. This is for one simple action, **its ability to increase blood and oxygen to the brain!**

Ginkgo has become famous for increasing memory and has been used effectively with Alzheimer's Disease patients. According to the American Medical Association, Ginkgo stops and even reverses symptoms of dementia.

Ginkgo has also been found to improve tolerance to hypoxia (lack of oxygen to the brain.) Inhibit traumatic and chemically induced cerebral edema. Reduce retinal edema and cell damage to the retina. Inhibit age related reduction in brain chemicals. Increase memory capacity and learning performance. Improve blood flow in the small cerebral capillaries and destroy free radicals and hundreds of other health benefiting discoveries.

The current fad in herbal medicine with herbalists, and especially herbal product manufacturers, is to try to identify the "key" or "active ingredient" in an herb, then isolate it, concentrate it and make a standardized extract. "Active ingredient" is just a hip herbal word for a drug. What do they think, that God did a sloppy job and threw a bunch of garbage in with the few good chemicals, where is their faith? Nature is truly perfection.

Anyway, the scientific research backs up my faith because every time medical doctors try to isolate **Ginkgo Biloba leaf's** so-called active ingredients, the extract doesn't work. When will they get it: the herb, the whole herb and nothing but the whole herb! In fact, it has now been reported by the medical researchers that, *"the mechanism of action of Ginkgo biloba extract in the central nervous system is only partially understood, but the main effects seem to be related to its antioxidant properties, <u>which REQUIRE the synergistic action of the flavonoids, the terpenoids, ginkgolides, bilobalide, organic acids . . .</u>"* in other words all of the phytochemical constituents in the herbs. This again mirrors my clinical experience because isolated, standardized herbal tonics, no matter how potent and powerful their advertising was, DID NOT GET MY PATIENTS WELL, but the whole plant extracts that I made did!

The prestigous medical book, the *Merck Manual*, lists Ginkgo as therapeutic for Cerebral Vascular insufficiency.

Habanero peppers. Everything the scientific and medical research discovered about Ginkgo's miraculous healing ability is true, but in the clinic when I mixed it with Cayenne, WOW, it worked 100 times better. Remember, there is only one herb that when you ingest it, your face turns red. That's blood being forced to your head and I can't think of a more powerful herb to complement Ginkgo than one that BLASTS it up into your head and brain. **Rosemary leaf** and **flower** and **Kola nut** are famous and powerful cerebral stimulants that compliment the actions of Ginkgo and Cayenne.

DOSAGE

2 droppersful (30-60 drops) three times daily.

For price and quantity information please refer to your American Botanical Pharmacy 2001 Herbal Product Catalog or call 1-800-HERBDOC for your FREE copy.

DR. SCHULZE'S NERVE FORMULA

BOTANICAL INGREDIENTS **Valerian root**, *Valeriana officinales*, **Lobelia seed pods**, *Lobelia inflata*, **Passionflower herb**, *Passiflora incarnata*, **Hops flower**, *Humulus lupulus*, **Black Cohosh root**, *Cimicifuga racemosa*, **Blue Cohosh root**, *Caulophyllum thalictroides*, **Skullcap herb**, *Scutellaria lateriflora*, **and Wild Yam rhizome**, *Dioscorea villosa root*.

METABOLIC ACTION AND BOTANICAL CHEMISTRY The herbs in this formula are quite famous for being powerful sedatives and antispasmodics. They will relax, sedate and relieve anxiety, nervous tension and muscle spasms. They are also very effective for insomnia, restlessness and a wonderful sleep aid. Although these herbs contain no narcotic ingredients, they are still famous for their potent ability to relax and induce rest and sleep. This formula is useful for all types of muscle and nervous system spasms and cramps including nervous trembling disorders, seizures, fits, spastic bowel and menstrual cramps.

The majority of the medical and scientific community have finally accepted **Valerian root** and **Passionflower herb** as pharmacologically active herbs. Even the esteemed *Merck Manual* lists their therapeutic category as sedative. I said earlier, preparations of these herbs along with **Hops flower** are prescribed by medical doctors and sold in drugstores throughout the world as sedatives and antispasmodics. **Lobelia seed** (See Lobelia), **Black Cohosh root, Blue Cohosh root, Skullcap herb** and **Wild Yam** all hold esteem in traditional American Indian and Early American herbal medicine as sedative and antispasmodic plants.

DOSAGE

2 droppersful (30-60 drops) three to four times daily. Up to 4 droppersful may be used as needed, more in an emergency.

Don't forget, B-Vitamins and B-Vitamin Complex nutrients are the fuel that your entire nervous system runs on and constantly needs to repair itself. This is why I made every patient on the **Nerve Formula** take a double dose of **SuperFood** which is the highest natural source of B-Vitamins available.

For price and quantity information please refer to your American Botanical Pharmacy 2001 Herbal Product Catalog or call 1-800-HERBDOC for your FREE copy.

DR. SCHULZE'S LOBELIA TINCTURE

BOTANICAL INGREDIENTS *Lobelia seeds, Lobelia inflata, in a base of Organic, Unfiltered, Raw Apple Cider Vinegar and Grain Alcohol.*

METABOLIC ACTION AND BOTANICAL CHEMISTRY Alkaloids are considered to be one of the most powerful types of chemicals found in plants. Not all plants have them and those that do may contain only one or two. Lobelia contains fourteen known alkaloids, the most prominent being lobeline! This may be why it has so many actions and uses and does so many different things. Many herbal doctors feel that it synergistically helps your body do whatever it needs to do. In the esteemed *Merck Manual* (the American book of chemicals) it lists Lobelia as an expectorant. It is famous for being able to purge mucous, fluid, and just about anything from the lungs. It also dilates the bronchial tubes which makes expectoration and breathing easier thus it was often referred to as Asthma weed, because so many asthmatics use it to literally stay alive. It is sold today in drugstores and pharmacies around the world, but not in the United States. I say it is also an expectorant to the whole body. If a very high dose is taken, you will experience a whole body purge, where you urinate, sweat, vomit and even poop, often all at the same time. Maybe more important than anything, in the clinic I have seen it work miracles by acting as a whole body relaxant and antispasmodic when nothing else seemed to work. Many herbalists, including Dr. Christopher and now myself, saw that it seemed to open up the body, make the body more available for herbs, juices, whatever and make everything work better. This is one herb that must be experienced and ALWAYS kept in your Herbal Emergency Kit.

DOSAGE

For bronchial dilation and antispasmodic action five or more drops is a good starting dose. More can be used but this is a powerful herb, so work your way up in dosage slowly. Many of my patients used 2 droppersful as their average dosage.

For price and quantity information please refer to your American Botanical Pharmacy 2001 Herbal Product Catalog or call 1-800-HERBDOC for your FREE copy.

DR. SCHULZE'S SUPERFOOD

BOTANICAL INGREDIENTS *Spirulina Blue-Green Algae, Chlorella Algae, Alfalfa grass, Barley grass, Wheat grass, Purple Dulse Seaweed, Beet root, Spinach leaf, Rose hips, Orange and Lemon peels and non-active Saccharomyces cervisiae Nutritional Yeast.*

METABOLIC ACTION AND BOTANICAL CHEMISTRY A lack of nutrition in your blood can cause everything from low energy and a weak immune system to virtually any disease. Your speed and ability to recover are greatly reduced when you are nutritionally depleted. Nutrition is what builds every cell, every organ and every metabolic chemical in your body. **Nutrition is what builds your body; it's what YOU are made out of.**

God and Nature have blessed us with certain foods and herbs that are so nutritionally potent, concentrated and complete, I call them the SUPERFOODS. This perfectly balanced blend of SUPERFOODS will supply you with a wide range of natural food source vitamins, minerals, amino acids and essential trace nutrients. It's a Natural Blood Transfusion.

We are currently entering a new era of nutrition. It is no longer a matter of how many milligrams you take of this or that nutrient, but how much of what you are taking is actually ending up in your bloodstream and getting to the organs that need it.

I designed and developed **SUPERFOOD** using numerous single-celled microplants. What this means in plain English is that you can assimilate it in minutes, right into your blood: where you need it.

Spirulina Blue-Green Algae has been discovered to be one of the most concentrated, nutritious foods on the planet. We use the only organically grown Spirulina in the world, from Hawaii. The high amount of sunshine there makes this spirulina higher in Beta-Carotene and the numerous other carotenoids than any other. It is also a rich source of B-Vitamins, especially B-12, and the highest natural source of complete protein known (75%). Grown using water pumped from 2000 feet deep in the ocean, this Spirulina is also one of the richest sources of minerals anywhere.

Chlorella, another blue-green algae, is also an extremely concentrated source of nutrition and complements Spirulina well. While all the nutritionists argue over which one is better to use, Spirulina or Chlorella, I put them both in my SUPERFOOD formula. This is simply because my focus is not to win a nutritional argument, but to help you get healthy, period.

Alfalfa, Barley & Wheat Grasses are literally Nature's most potent and complete vitamin and mineral herbs. They are mildly cleansing and the greatest sources of nutrition of any grasses. Grain grasses are more potent than the grains themselves, offering us a rich array of vitamins, minerals and chlorophyll.

Purple Dulse Seaweed Seaweeds are the richest source of assimilable minerals on the planet. They contain all the minerals and trace minerals that are found in the oceans and in the earth's crust. We chose Purple Scandinavian Dulse because it has the highest mineral concentration, but also tastes bland. Many seaweeds taste very fishy; dulse does not.

Beet Root & Spinach Leaf are some of the richest, most assimilable sources of organic minerals, especially iron. Beets, being a root vegetable and growing underground, change inorganic hard rock mineral elements into plant minerals that are digestible by us. Spinach is a rich source of calcium, iron, and vitamin K. Both of these plants are famous for their blood building abilities.

Rose Hips, Orange and Lemon Peels are revered as some of the best sources of vitamin C. These fruits are also a balanced C-complex source. The citrus peels contain bioflavinoids, rutin, hesperidin, calcium and all of the trace elements that are now known to be necessary to assimilate vitamin C.

Non-Active Saccharomyces Cervisiae Nutritional Yeast is grown on beets and pure molasses and literally vacuums all the B-vitamins out of whatever it is grown on. It is the second highest source of complete protein in nature, (50%), and the richest source of B vitamins ever found. It is also a rich source of iron and numerous other minerals. The yeast we choose is heated just high enough to absolutely destroy any yeast activity, but not high enough to lessen the B Vitamin content. It is totally NON-ACTIVE and safe for any patient with candida albicans or on yeast-free diets.

DOSAGE

Two rounded tablespoons of **SUPERFOOD**, added to your favorite juice or blender drink, gives you two to five times of most vitamins you need for the entire day. What's even better is that you can assimilate these foods so easily, the nutrients can enter your bloodstream going to work within fifteen minutes. If you are not used to nutritional drinks, then for the first week use only 1 tablespoon of **SUPERFOOD**, and work your way up to 2 tablespoons.

SUGGESTED SUPERFOOD DRINK: A perfect way to start your day: In a blender mix 8 ounces of fresh apple juice, 8 ounces of pure water, 1 banana or 1/2 cup of fresh fruit, and 2 tablespoons of **SUPERFOOD** Vitamin and Mineral Supplement. Follow this program for 30 days and feel and see the difference in your life.
This is a Vegan/Vegetarian Product. NO Animal Ingredients. SUPERFOOD is tested on animals only if they volunteer, and they love it.

For price and quantity information please refer to your American Botanical Pharmacy 2001 Herbal Product Catalog or call 1-800-HERBDOC for your FREE copy.

> *"The healing journey you're about to embark on is not a burden or a chore, but a blessing. It will be your greatest adventure inward to discover and create a new life, a new you."*
> *- Dr. Richard Schulze*

CHAPTER 9

LUNG DISORDERS

EXPLANATION OF SYSTEM

Your lungs are the largest organs located in the thorax. Your right lung consists of the upper, middle, and lower lobes. Your left lung consists of an upper and a lower lobe. Your lungs touch the heart on both sides.

Your lungs exchange carbon dioxide for oxygen in the blood. In the lung, oxygen-poor blood that enters the heart from the veins is supplied with fresh oxygen, and carbon dioxide is removed in a process called gas exchange. The trachea, or windpipe, and bronchi are the passageways for air to enter and leave the lungs. The lungs are lined with a membrane called the pleura that secretes a substance that reduces the friction caused by movement of the lungs during breathing.

The trachea branches into the left and right primary bronchi. One bronchi enters the left lung, and the other, the right lung. The bronchi further branch irregularly, narrowing gradually until they reach the bronchioles and, finally, the alveoli, where gases are exchanged. Alveoli are round sac-like structures that fill with air upon inhalation. There are approximately 600 million alveoli. 75% of the round surface of an alveolus is covered by tiny blood vessels called capillaries.

Upon breathing in (inhalation), air high in oxygen enters the lungs where it travels down to the alveoli. The oxygen crosses over (in a process called diffusion) into the capillaries. The capillaries join together and become larger and larger arteries until they become the pulmonary veins which take this oxygen-rich blood back to the heart to be pumped to the rest of the body. At the same time, the capillaries containing oxygen-poor blood high in carbon dioxide dump their carbon dioxide into the alveoli to be removed when a person breathes out (exhales). A person cannot completely exhale; there is always some air left in the lungs after exhalation. The presence of this residual air in the alveoli makes it easier to reexpand them with air on the next inhalation.

Inhalation occurs when the diaphragm contracts which causes the chest to expand. The diaphragm is a large dome-shaped muscle which separates the abdomen from the chest cavity, curving downward. It contracts with each inhalation, flattening out downward, allowing the bottoms of the lungs to descend. Because of the expansion of the chest on inhalation, the pressure inside the lungs decreases forming a vacuum which sucks air into the lungs. The intercostal muscles also help in expanding the chest. They are located between the ribs. (inter = between, costal = ribs) The diaphragm relaxes with each exhalation, raising itself back up and restoring its downward curving shape (like an upside down bowl) forcing the air back out of your lungs.

GLOSSARY OF PULMONARY SYSTEM TERMINOLOGY

Alveoli air cells of the lungs

Arterial blood gas test whereby blood is withdrawn from an artery in the wrist to analyze the amount of oxygen and carbon dioxide in the blood to determine how well the lungs are functioning; common test for COPD

Asthma disease caused by an over sensitivity of the trachea and bronchi, causing them to constrict which produces shortness of breath and wheezing.

Bronchoalveolar carcinoma type of lung cancer

Bronchitis inflammation of the mucous membrane of the bronchial airways, causing coughing and increased mucous secretions from the bronchioles. Acute bronchitis usually follows a viral infection, and chronic bronchitis is most often caused by smoking.

Bronchoscopy procedure during which an instrument (bronchoscope) is inserted through the windpipe into the bronchial tubes to examine and collect specimens from the bronchi

Bronchus one of the two large branches of the trachea (windpipe)

Chest X-ray an x-ray of the chest, usually showing abnormalities of the lungs, heart, ribs, and spine

COPD chronic obstructive pulmonary disease

Corticosteroids medication that suppresses the immune system, used to treat some lung diseases caused by an overactive immune system

Emphysema chronic pulmonary disease marked by an abnormal increase in the size of air spaces. Symptoms include shortness of breath, and increased effort to breathe, over the long term causing an enlarged chest (barrel chest.)

Lung biopsy surgical procedure whereby lung tissue is cut out to be tested for certain diseases such as cancer, infection, etc.

Lung cancer	types include small cell carcinoma, large cell carcinoma, bronchoalveolar carcinoma, adenocarcinoma, and squamous cell carcinoma. Symptoms include cough. Patients commonly cough up blood-streaked sputum.
Nebulizer	device for producing a fine spray or mist that when inhaled, delivers liquid medication to the lungs
Pleura	thin membrane that surrounds the lungs
Pleurisy	inflammation of the pleura; usually associated with autoimmune disorders such as lupus; also called pleuritis
Pneumonia	inflammation of the alveoli, interstitial tissue, and bronchioles of the lungs due to infection by bacteria, viruses, or other infectious organisms, or to irritation by chemicals or other agents. These normally air-filled tissues fill with fluid causing difficulty with breathing.
Pneumothorax	collection of air or gas in the pleural space that lines the lungs
Pulmonary	concerning or involving the lungs
Pneumoconiosis	an occupational lung disease caused by the long term inhalation of dust particles such as in mining or stonecutting. Advanced cases lead to scarring and severe impairment of breathing, eventually leading to death.
Sputum	substance expelled by coughing or clearing the throat containing material from the respiratory tract such as cells, mucous, blood, pus, and microorganisms
Sputum analysis	analysis of a patient's sputum to test for infection, cancer, and other lung diseases
Steroids	see corticosteroids
Thoracentesis	surgical puncture of the chest for removal and draining of fluids in the lungs; usually using a large-bore needle. A complication of this procedure is collapse of the lung.
Thoracotomy	surgical incision of the chest wall

Tuberculosis	also called TB. A highly infectious and contagious disease of the lungs caused by a bacteria called *mycobacterium tuberculosis* which causes inflammation, scarring, calcification and death of lung tissue. Diagnosed by a tuberculin skin test (called a TB skin test) and chest x-rays.

SPECIFIC HERBAL FORMULAE FOR THE LUNGS

DR. SCHULZE'S LOBELIA TINCTURE

BOTANICAL INGREDIENTS *Lobelia seeds, Lobelia inflata,* **in a base of Organic, Unfiltered, Raw Apple Cider Vinegar and Grain Alcohol.**

METABOLIC ACTION AND BOTANICAL CHEMISTRY Alkaloids are considered to be one of the most powerful types of chemicals found in plants. Not all plants have them and those that do may contain only one or two. Lobelia contains fourteen known alkaloids, the most prominent being lobeline! This may be why it has so many actions and uses and does so many different things. Many herbal doctors feel that it synergistically helps your body do whatever it needs to do. In the esteemed *Merck Manual* (the American book of chemicals) it lists Lobelia as an expectorant. It is famous for being able to purge mucous, fluid, and just about anything from the lungs. It also dilates the bronchial tubes which makes expectoration and breathing easier thus it was often referred to as Asthma weed, because so many asthmatics use it to literally stay alive. It is sold today in drugstores and pharmacies around the world, but not in the United States. I say it is also an expectorant to the whole body. If a very high dose is taken, you will experience a whole body purge, where you urinate, sweat, vomit and even poop, often all at the same time. Maybe more important than anything, in the clinic I have seen it work miracles by acting as a whole body relaxant and antispasmodic when nothing else seemed to work. Many herbalists, including Dr. Christopher and now myself, saw that it seemed to open up the body, make the body more available for herbs, juices, whatever and make everything work better. This is one herb that must be experienced and ALWAYS kept in your Herbal Emergency Kit.

DOSAGE
For bronchial dilation and antispasmodic action five or more drops is a good starting dose. More can be used but this is a powerful herb, so work your way up in dosage slowly. Many of my patients used 2 droppersful as their average dosage.

For price and quantity information please refer to your American Botanical Pharmacy 2001 Herbal Product Catalog or call 1-800-HERBDOC for your FREE copy.

DR. SCHULZE'S SINUS/LUNG FORMULA

BOTANICAL INGREDIENTS *Ma Huang,* *Ephedra species,* **Lobelia seed and pod,** *Lobelia inflata,* **Kola nut,** *Cola acuminata,* **Coffee bean,** *Coffee arabica,* **Licorice root,** *Glycyrrhiza Glabra,* **Star Anise,** *Illicium verum,* **Fennel seed,** *Foeniculum officinale,* **Thyme leaf,** *Thymus vulgaris,* **Peppermint leaf and Peppermint essential oils,** *Mentha piperita.*

METABOLIC ACTION AND BOTANICAL CHEMISTRY There are many types of phytochemicals (plant chemicals.) One of the most powerful groups of these chemicals is called alkaloids. Common plant alkaloids that you may have heard of are caffeine, morphine, dexedrine; so you see these are very strong plant chemicals. **Ma Huang – Ephedra** contains the powerful alkaloids ephedrine and pseudoephedrine which have a strong antihistamine and vasoconstrictor effect. **Lobelia seed and pod,** contains fourteen known alkaloids. One of these alkaloids, Lobeline, is a powerful dilator to the bronchial tubes that are the entry way to your lungs. Lobelia also is an expectorant and antispasmodic. These two herbs together help reduce the symptoms of allergic reactions, cold and the flu, and also help drain, open up, expel mucous and in turn dry up the sinus and clear the lungs. Even the esteemed medical/chemical text the Merck Index lists Ephedra as a Decongestant and Bronchial Dilator and also lists Lobelia as an Expectorant. **Kola nut and Coffee bean** both contain the alkaloid caffeine which stimulates your body to produce more adrenaline or epinephrine. This natural body chemical dilates the bronchial tubes, relieves asthma attacks and eases breathing. The vapors of **Peppermint's** essential oils are antispasmodic and relieve excess coughing.

DOSAGE
1-2 droppersful as needed, dilute in a few ounces of water or juice.
FDA WARNING: Do not exceed 8 droppersful in one day.

<u>**CAUTION:**</u> This formula contains naturally occurring ephedrine, lobeline and caffeine, three very powerful alkaloids. Do not use if you are pregnant or nursing or have any disease. Generally this formula should not be used after 6 p.m. unless sleep is unlikely due to breathing difficulty.

For price and quantity information please refer to your American Botanical Pharmacy 2001 Herbal Product Catalog or call 1-800-HERBDOC for your FREE copy.

DR. SCHULZE'S SUPERTONIC

BOTANICAL INGREDIENTS *Fresh juices of Organic Habanero Cayenne, Capsicum annum,* **Organic Garlic,** *Allium sativum,* **Organic Onion,** *Allium cepa,* **Organic Ginger,** *Zingiber officinale,* **Organic Horseradish,** *Armoracia rusticana,* **and Organic Raw Unfiltered Apple Cider Vinegar.**

METABOLIC ACTION AND BOTANICAL CHEMISTRY Garlic is a broad spectrum antibiotic, destroying both gram-positive and gram-negative bacteria. Unlike chemical antibiotics that kill off the millions of *friendly* bacteria that your body needs, Garlic only kills the *bad guys* and even promotes and increases your healthy bacteria. It is also a very potent, anti-viral which really makes it a specific for colds, influenza and upper respiratory infections. Garlic is also a powerful anti-fungal and literally destroys any antigen, pathogen and any harmful or disease causing micro-organism that can hurt you. **Onion** is Garlic's next of kin and has a similar but milder action. Together they are a killing duo. **Horseradish** is a potent herb for the sinus and lungs. It opens the sinus passages and increases the circulation there, where, most doctors agree, the common cold and influenza often starts. **Cayenne** and **Ginger** are like a nuclear blast to your body's circulation. This powerful tag team will unblock anything, anywhere!

So just imagine, you have the two strongest herbs to kill EVERY germ known and the three most powerful herbs to blast them around your entire body. It doesn't get any better. That's the bottom line.

DOSAGE

1-4 droppersful in a shot glass. First timers may want to mix this dosage half and half with water. Whether you dilute it or take it straight, gargle with it for a minute and then swallow.

As you can imagine, this is a strong and powerful tonic and has a taste to match. Actually, it also happens to be the world's greatest tasting salad dressing when mixed with a little virgin olive oil. The following is my personal favorite way to take it: In a shot glass or small cup, put 3 or 4 droppersful of SuperTonic and 8 droppersful of Echinacea Plus. Add about an ounce of fresh squeezed apple juice. Gargle and swallow. I do this about every hour when I feel out of sorts. In the clinic, this kept me going when my sickest patients were coughing, sneezing and even vomiting on me.

There are a million more ways to use it, straight or diluted. I welcome your personal favorites. After all, 98% of what I know I learned from my patients and you, my customers.

For price and quantity information please refer to your American Botanical Pharmacy 2001 Herbal Product Catalog or call 1-800-HERBDOC for your FREE copy.

CHAPTER 10

THE SKIN

EXPLANATION OF SYSTEM

The skin which covers all the surfaces of the body is the largest organ of the body. Its weight makes up approximately 8.8% of total body weight. The skin provides protection against heat, cold, sun rays, friction, pressure and various chemicals. It also contains sense receptors that sense pain, touch and temperature. The skin has an acid pH which is a defense against certain microorganisms.

Skin is composed of an outer layer called the epidermis and an inner layer called the dermis. The subcutaneous tissue (sub = beneath, cutaneous = skin) lies beneath the surface of the skin and includes such structures as the sweat glands, sebaceous glands, hair roots and follicles, blood vessels, lymphatic vessels, and peripheral nerves.

Sebaceous glands secrete an oily substance called sebum at the base of the hair roots to cover the surface of the hair and skin with an oily film. Apocrine sweat glands produce a complex secretion with a strong odor. They are found in highest concentration in certain areas of the body, such as in the arm pits and in the genital region. Eccrine sweat glands are distributed throughout the entire epidermis and are concentrated mainly in the palms of the hands and the soles of the feet. The production of sweat helps the body to adjust its internal temperature. Sweat cools the body by evaporation and rids it of waste through the pores of the skin. It contains waste products such as urea, as well as salts and fatty substances. The amount of sweat produced daily is about a liter, and in hot conditions may be as much as 10-15 liters in 24 hours.

Melanin is the pigment found in the skin that is responsible for hair and skin color. It is produced by cells called melanocytes found in the lower epidermis, and migrates towards the epidermis. The skin color varies according to the amount of melanin in the cells. Exposure to sunlight stimulates melanin production to cause a "tan". Moles are areas of concentrated melanin.

GLOSSARY OF DERMATOLOGIC TERMINOLOGY

Allergic dermatitis   inflammation of the skin caused by an allergy to a certain substance such as nickel, etc.

Basal cell carcinoma   type of skin cancer

Contact dermatitis   inflammation of the skin caused by contact with an irritant such as poison ivy, soaps, perfumes, and other chemicals

Cyst   closed sac or pouch, with a definite wall, that contains fluid, semifluid, or solid material; usually an abnormal structure resulting from abnormal development, blocked ducts, or parasite infection

Dermatology   science of the skin and its diseases

Dermatitis   inflammation of the skin causing itching, redness, and various skin lesions

Eczema   an acute or chronic skin inflammation with redness, red bumps, fluid-filled bumps, pus-filled bumps, scales, crusts, or scabs alone or in combination; usually occuring in allergic patients

Epidermis   outermost layer of the skin

Follicle   small sac or cavity that secretes substances

Hives   common name for urticaria. A sudden eruption of raised pale wheals which are associated with severe itching. They may be caused by an allergy or contact with external irritants such as insect bites, pollen, foods, medications or stress.

Lesion   circumscribed area of pathologically altered tissue

Melanoma   cancerous, darkly pigmented mole or tumor of the skin caused by excessive exposure to the sun. The most dangerous type of skin cancer which easily spreads to distant areas of the body.

Pemphigus   acute or chronic autoimmune disease marked by the occurrence of large fluid-filled blisters that appear and disappear suddenly

Psoriasis   chronic skin disease marked by raised red areas which join together and eventually develop white scales on top, frequently located on the scalp, knees, elbows, belly button and genitals

Punch biopsy   procedure during which an instrument is used to punch a small circular hole in the skin to test the skin for diseases

Pustule   small raised area of the skin filled with pus

Rosacea   chronic disease of the skin of the face usually occurring in middle-aged and older persons; marked by varying degrees of red bumps, pus-filled bumps, redness, dilated blood vessels, and enlargement of the nose tissue

Sebaceous cyst   cyst of the sebaceous gland

Sebaceous gland gland in the skin that secretes an oil called sebum; most open into hair follicles, lubricating the hair shaft

Squamous cell carcinoma type of skin cancer; usually invades and spreads locally (not to distant areas), commonly on the face, causing severe disfigurement and death if left untreated

Subcutaneous   beneath the skin

Vesicle   raised area of the skin filled with clear fluid as in herpes infections

Wart   circumscribed elevation of the skin resulting from overgrowth of the epidermis; caused by a papilloma virus

SPECIFIC HERBAL FORMULAE FOR THE SKIN

DR. SCHULZE'S JOJOBA & TEA TREE OIL

BOTANICAL INGREDIENTS *Organic Jojoba oil and Organic 9% Tea Tree oil, Melaeuca alternifolia.*

METABOLIC ACTION AND BOTANICAL CHEMISTRY For hundreds of years sperm whale oil was prized for its many uses. Its high ester content made it an unique oil that would actually deeply penetrate the skin and not only soften it but soothe it (emollient). But this oil is made from killing and butchering whales. As I have always said, there is an herbal replacement for everything from the animal kingdom and the days of needing shark fins, bear gallbladders, tiger penises, rhinoceros horn, snake gall bladders and even whale oil are over, THERE IS ALWAYS AN HERBAL REPLACEMENT!

Jojoba oil (pronounced ho-ho ba) is made from the bean of a desert plant. It is extremely high in these similar esters and it is DEEPLY penetrating, soothing and healing to the skin. Other plant oils when applied to the skin mostly just smear around and sit on the surface. On the contrary, Jojoba penetrates all layers of the skin which also makes it a great catalyst to help other oils it is mixed with to penetrate. Jojoba oil is also naturally SPF (sun protection factor) 16 which makes it an excellent sunscreen.

Tea Tree oil is made from a shrub native to Australia. It has been used widely in traditional herbal medicine but fell out of popularity since WWII, you guessed it again, when antibiotics were touted as a cure-all for everything. It is now enjoying an herbal renaissance and this very potent oil contains volatile oils that are highly antibacterial and anti-fungal at concentrations of only 1% to 2%. I found in the clinic that when I took its concentration up to 9%, it was even more effective, but still mild enough for the tenderest of babies' bottoms and the genitals.

DOSAGE
One or more droppersful rubbed well into the skin. Use as needed. Don't limit yourself.

For price and quantity information please refer to your American Botanical Pharmacy 2001 Herbal Product Catalog or call 1-800-HERBDOC for your FREE copy.

CHAPTER 11

HEARING AND EYESIGHT

EXPLANATION OF SYSTEM

THE EAR

The ear governs hearing and balance. It includes the outer cartilage known as the pinna, the auditory organs, and the vestibula organs (balance).

Sound waves pass from the outside through the external auditory meatus to the eardrum, a thin membrane which receives the vibrations. Just behind the eardrum are three bones called the hammer, anvil and stapes which magnify the vibrations. Then, the vibrations pass to the inner ear where they go through the scala vestibuli, the scala tympani, and the cochlea. The vibrations are changed into electric signals in the hair cells in the organ of Corti located inside the cochlea. These signals are then transmitted to the auditory nerve which relays the signals to the brain to be interpreted as sounds.

Next to the cochlea are the organs of balance – the utricle, saccule, and semicircular ducts. A fluid called endolymph fills the semicircular ducts and moves when the head is turned. Movement of the fluid stimulates the hair cells inside to move which sends signals to the vestibular nerves concerning rotation and balance. Finally, these nerves transmit signals to the brain.

The inner ear is connected to the pharynx by way of the auditory tube, also called the Eustachian tube. When there is a large change in pressure, such as what happens in high altitudes (on airplanes or in the mountains) the semicircular ducts cannot handle the change in air pressure inside and outside the eardrum quickly enough. The pressures can be equalized by yawning or swallowing, which opens the entrance of the Eustachian tube. Blockage of the Eustachian tube leads to infection of the middle ear (called otitis media).

THE EYE

The eyeball, cushioned in a layer of fat, is located inside a protective socket within the skull. The eyeball is made up of two spheres. The first one is the largest, and is the first thing we notice when looking at an eyeball. This large sphere is called the posterior chamber (vitreous chamber) and is covered on all sides by the sclera (we know it as the "white" of the eye). The second much smaller sphere is attached to and lies in the front of the eyeball. It is called the anterior chamber of the eye, which is covered by the cornea. There are three pairs of muscles which control the movement of the eyeball (extraocular muscles.) They allow us to look up, down, and in all other directions.

Tears are produced in the lacrimal gland which lies above the eyeball and towards the direction of the ear. Tears have an acid pH which protects the eye from invasion by microorganisms. From the lacrimal gland, tears flow through ducts to the eye to wet the surface of the eyeball. Tears then pass downward from the inner corner of the eye into the lacrimal punctum and tear sac and through the lower nasal passage. When crying, more tears than usual drain down these ducts into the nose which explains why people get a runny nose when they cry.

Vision can be easily understood by looking at the eye like a camera. Visual information enters through the pupil in the form of light. The cornea is the clear rounded portion of the eye which covers the pupil and the iris (the colored portion of the eye). It is clear so that light can pass through it. The iris contracts and relaxes to let the proper amount of light in, depending on the environment. In this way, it is like the aperture of a camera. The light goes through the lens of the eye which bends the light rays in a certain way so that they come to a focus on the back of the eyeball. The lens is flexible and can change its thickness to focus on far away as well as nearby objects. In this way, the lens of the eye corresponds to the lens of a camera. The light hits the back of the eyeball which is lined with a special light-sensitive membrane called the retina. The retina is to the eyeball what film is to the camera. The retina contains special receptor cells (called rods) which are responsible for sensing changes in light, and the cones (which sense colors.) The exact spot where most of the light rays hit is called the macula. This area contains the highest concentration of cones and is responsible for sight in the center of the visual field, and for discriminating fine details. The images are projected onto the retina and changed to electric signals which are sent to the brain via the optic nerve for interpretation as color and objects. (This would be like getting your pictures developed at the photo shop.) The rods and cones and other visual cells are all connected to a nerve fiber which combine to form the optic nerve. The optic nerve connects the back of the eyeball to the brain.

GLOSSARY OF AUDITORY AND OPTIC TERMINOLOGY

Auditory   pertaining to the sense of hearing

Cataract   dulling and opaqueness of the lens of the eye which is normally transparent, causing progressive blurring of the vision

Cochlea   winding cone-shaped tube forming a portion of the inner ear; it contains the organ of Corti, the receptor for hearing

Conjunctiva   mucous membrane that lines the eyelids and is reflected
                         onto the eyeball

Conjunctivitis   inflammation or infection of the conjunctiva, usually caused by
                         allergies or microorganisms. Infectious conjunctivitis is highly
                         contagious, and is commonly called "pink eye".

Cornea   transparent frontal portion of the fibrous outer layer of the eyeball

External   canal which carries sound waves from the outside of the head
auditory meatus   to the eardrum

Glaucoma   group of eye diseases characterized by increased intraocular pressure,
                         resulting in atrophy of the optic nerve and possible blindness

Hyperopia   also called farsightedness; difficulty with or inability to see close up
                         objects

Iris   round colored portion of the eye that surrounds the pupil

Macular   degeneration of the macular area of the retina of the eye which is an
Degeneration   area important in the visualization of fine details; leads to loss
                         of sight in the center of the field of vision

Myopia   also called nearsightedness; difficulty with or inability to see far
                         away objects.

Ocular   pertaining to the eye or vision

Ophthalmoscope lighted instrument used to examine the interior of the eye such as
                         the lens and the retina

Otitis externa   infection of the outer ear canal; also called "swimmer's ear."

Otitis interna   infection of the inner ear containing the labyrinths; also called
                         labyrinthitis; symptoms include dizziness

Otitis media   presence of fluid in the middle ear and signs of infection such as
                         fever, irritability, drainage from the ear, ear pain, and sometimes
                         temporary hearing loss

Presbyopia   condition caused by advancing age in which the lens loses its
                         flexibility and thickens, causing difficulty in focusing on nearby objects

Pterygium	triangular thickening of the conjunctiva extending from the inner corner of the eye to the border of the cornea and sometimes extending onto the cornea, interfering with vision
Pupil	black, round opening at the center of the iris of the eye which contracts when exposed to bright light to let in less light and expands in the dark to let in more light
Retina	light-sensitive innermost layer of the eyeball which receives images transmitted through the lens and contains the receptors for vision, the rods and cones
Retinitis Pigmentosa	chronic progressive eye disease beginning in childhood in which the retina deteriorates, the optic nerve atrophies, and pigments appear in the retina causing loss of vision in the periphery, (tunnel vision); disease progresses to total blindness
Sclera	the "whites" of the eyes
Semicircular ducts	one of the passages of the inner ear concerned with detecting motion
Tympanic membrane	the eardrum

SPECIFIC HERBAL FORMULAE FOR HEARING AND EYESIGHT

DR. SCHULZE'S EYEBRIGHT FORMULA

BOTANICAL INGREDIENTS *Eyebright herb and flower, Euphrasia officinales,* **Goldenseal root,** *Hydrastis Canadensis,* **Rue flower,** *Ruta graveolens,* **Mullein flower,** *Verbascum thapsus,* **Fennel seed,** *Foeniculum officinale,* **Red Raspberry leaf,** *Rubus idaeus* **and Cayenne,** *Capsicum annum.*

METABOLIC ACTION AND BOTANICAL CHEMISTRY Goldenseal root is famous for being a mild acting, but highly effective antibacterial and antiseptic herb. In the clinic I found it extremely useful for destroying infection around the sensitive areas of the body like the eyes, inside the sinus, and sensitive mucous membrane areas where garlic could be too strong. It contains the alkaloids hydrastine, berberine and canadine, and volatile oils and resins. The first two alkaloids are listed medically as antibacterial and antiseptic.

Eyebright and **Fennel** both have a long history of use for the eyes, soothing inflammation and reducing irritation, especially for conjunctivitis. **Mullein** is very soothing and demulcent to the delicate mucous membranes. **Red Raspberry** is a mild astringent and **Rue** an antispasmodic. The law restricts me from commenting any further.

DOSAGE
Mix 2 to 10 drops of the tincture into 1 ounce of room temperature distilled water. It is illegal for me to suggest putting it into your eyes.

For price and quantity information please refer to your American Botanical Pharmacy 2001 Herbal Product Catalog or call 1-800-HERBDOC for your FREE copy.

DR. SCHULZE'S BRAIN FORMULA

BOTANICAL INGREDIENTS *Ginkgo Biloba leaf,* Ginkgo biloba, **Rosemary leaf and flower,** Rosmarinus officinale, **Kola nut,** Cola acuminata **and Cayenne peppers,** Capsicum annum.

METABOLIC ACTION AND BOTANICAL CHEMISTRY Ginkgo has also been found to improve tolerance to hypoxia (lack of oxygen to the brain.) Inhibit traumatic and chemically induced cerebral edema. Reduce retinal edema and cell damage to the retina. Inhibit age related reduction in brain chemicals. Increase memory capacity and learning performance. Improve blood flow in the small cerebral capillaries and destroy free radicals and hundreds of other health benefiting discoveries.

Ginkgo has been proven effective for hearing and eyesight problems, tinnitis (ringing in the ear), vertigo (balance problems and dizziness), deafness and other inner ear problems. Many people using Ginkgo have experienced miraculous results with eyesight problems. For even more powerful results, use in conjunction with my **Eyebright Formula.**

The current fad in herbal medicine with herbalists, and especially herbal product manufacturers, is to try to identify the "key" or "active ingredient" in an herb, then isolate it, concentrate it and make a standardized extract. "Active ingredient" is just a hip herbal word for a drug. What do they think, that God did a sloppy job and threw a bunch of garbage in with the few good chemicals, where is their faith? Nature is truly perfection.

Anyway, the scientific research backs up my faith because every time medical doctors try to isolate **Ginkgo Biloba leaf's** so-called active ingredients, the extract doesn't work. When will they get it: the herb, the whole herb and nothing but the whole herb! In fact, it has now been reported by the medical researchers that, "the mechanism of action of Ginkgo biloba extract in the central nervous system is only partially understood, but the main effects seem to be related to its antioxidant properties, which REQUIRE the synergistic action of the flavonoids, the terpenoids, ginkgolides, bilobalide, organic acids . . ." in other words all of the phytochemical constituents in the herbs. This again mirrors my clinical experience because isolated, standardized herbal tonics, no matter how potent and powerful their advertising was, DID NOT GET MY PATIENTS WELL, but the whole plant extracts that I made did!

The prestigious medical book, the *Merck Manual,* lists Ginkgo as therapeutic for Cerebral Vascular insufficiency.

Habanero peppers. Everything the scientific and medical research discovered about Ginkgo's miraculous healing ability is true, but in the clinic when I mixed it with Cayenne, WOW, it worked 100 times better. Remember, there is only one herb that when you ingest it, your face turns red. That's blood being forced to your head and I can't think of a more powerful herb to complement Ginkgo than one that BLASTS it up into your head and brain. **Rosemary leaf** and **flower** and **Kola nut** are famous and powerful cerebral stimulants that compliment the actions of Ginkgo and Cayenne.

DOSAGE
2 droppersful (30-60 drops) three times daily.

For price and quantity information please refer to your American Botanical Pharmacy 2001 Herbal Product Catalog or call 1-800-HERBDOC for your FREE copy.

"If you are like me and you want to get started on your health and healing NOW, see the Special Deal I have put together on the next page.

So now you don't have to worry whether or not you are ordering the right thing. These are the foundational formulae that I started <u>every</u> patient on that came into my clinic regardless of what disease or illness they had."

- Dr. Richard Schulze

THE BEST PLACE TO START

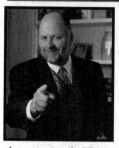

"IT'S LIKE BEING A PATIENT IN DR. SCHULZE'S CLINIC."

THIS IS WHERE TO START!

Remember, I know what it's like to be sick. And if you are searching for healing answers, I know everyone's got an opinion on what you should or shouldn't do. From running my clinic for so many years I also know that when you're sick, you comprehend less, you're foggier and get confused easier. This program is a no brainer, and I don't mean that as an insult. This is the exact program I gave to EVERY ONE of my patients that came to see me for a first visit in my clinic, EVERY SINGLE ONE OF THEM!

GET __MAXIMUM__ RESULTS!

This program is the foundation of good health that everyone needs. __It's the herbal formulae that give people the most dramatic, feel good results.__ In fact many people who use only the 3 formulae in this program find that the vast majority, if not all of their aches, pains and problems, are GONE! This is because over 90% of Americans suffer from one, if not all three of the problems that this program addresses and corrects: **#1**- a lack of super nutrition in your bloodstream, **#2**- too much accumulated toxic waste in the body and **#3**- a weak immune system.

WITH __MINIMUM__ EFFORT!

For two decades I operated my clinic in Hollywood and Malibu, CA. My patients were movie directors, producers, actors, actresses and models. They had no time, period. You can't find busier people, under more stress, living a faster paced and more hectic life. They had NO TIME and any program I put them on, at least in the beginning, had to be EASY, FAST and SIMPLE. This entire program only takes about 2 MINUTES A DAY to prepare and do. No inverted head stands, high enemas or complex herbal sitz baths here. You have to pay more for all of that fun stuff. This program is very simple, __all you have to do is swallow.__ It doesn't get much easier and quicker.

THE "WHERE DO I START?" SPECIAL DEAL!

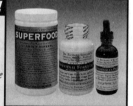

__SUPERFOOD__ *to supercharge your body with nutrition and give you more energy. Put two tablespoons in your morning drink, I don't care if its beer. SuperFood in beer is better than just beer.*

__INTESTINAL FORMULA #1__ *will clean you out, remove old waste and poison and keep you running smooth. Just swallow one pill after dinner. THAT'S IT!*

__ECHINACEA PLUS__ *to power up your immune system, to fight off what you have and increase your protection and resistance to what may be around the corner. Three or four times during the day just squirt 2 to 3 droppersful of this tonic into any drink you're drinking, or knock it back straight.*

I ASK YOU, DOES IT GET ANY EASIER?

What I guarantee: In a week you'll have more energy than you know what to do with; you'll feel better and more alive; you will be less sluggish and toxic; and a few of those problems you had, maybe all of them, well, they'll be gone.

SPECIAL PRICE $78.00

A BIOGRAPHY OF
DR. RICHARD SCHULZE

PERSONAL HEALING

When he was only 11 years old, his father died in his arms from a massive heart attack. At 14, his mother died of a heart attack. They were both only 55 yrs old.

At age 16 after a year of ill health, he was diagnosed by medical doctors to have a genetic heart deformity and deformed heart valves. The doctors said that unless he underwent open heart surgery immediately, he would be dead by the age of 20. This is because his weak deformed heart couldn't supply sufficient blood to an adult body.

He declined to have the surgery and instead made it his mission to discover alternative ways to heal his heart. After 3 years of numerous intensive natural healing programs and herbal formula, he was given a clean bill of health by the very surprised medical doctors. His heart was healed. After curing himself of this so-called *"incurable"* disease, through changes in his lifestyle and NO surgery, he then set out on a mission to help others. He enrolled himself into Naturopathic and Herbal College.

EDUCATION AND CREDENTIALS

Dr. Schulze studied with the famous European Naturopath, Paavo Airola. He trained and then served an internship with the famous natural healer Dr. Bernard Jensen. He also studied and apprenticed with *"America's greatest clinical herbalist"* the late Dr. John Christopher graduating to teach alongside him until his death. Besides having a Doctorate in Herbology and a Doctorate in Natural Medicine and 3 degrees in Iridology, he is certified in 8 different styles of Body Therapy and holds 3 black belts in the Martial Arts.

CLINICAL EXPERIENCE

In the early 1970's he opened his first Natural Healing Clinic in New York, and later in Southern California. He operated his natural healing clinic in America for almost 20 years, until his clinic was shut down. During this same time he also managed and directed other Natural Healing Clinics in Europe and Asia. In his two decades of practice he treated thousands of patients. In his second decade of clinical practice, he became famous for his intensive natural healing programs and his powerful herbal formulae.

His natural therapy programs and herbal formula are now used in clinics all over the world and have assisted an estimated hundred thousand people to create healing miracles and regain their health.

He is considered an innovator, a purist, even an extremist by many of his colleagues, but to his patients he was considered a life saver. Dr. Schulze always said, *"While Alternative doctors are pussy footing around trying to heal degenerative disease with aromatherapy and purple candles, the medical doctors are sharpening their knives, saws and drills, boiling down their chemotherapy and fine tuning their radiation beams. At least medical doctors know how to treat killer diseases, aggressively and with intensity."* In his clinic he was famous for his powerful and extreme natural healing programs and his potent clinical herbal formulae. He often said, *"I tried to kill my patients with the juicer, I tried to poison them with overdoses of strong herbal tonics, I tried to drown them in hydrotherapy, but the only thing that happened is that they got well. All the people I see dying and not recovering who are being treated with alternative medicine, are dying because they aren't doing enough. They need a natural healing blitz, turn the volume all the way up, and create a 24 hour a day natural healing lifestyle."*

Dr. Schulze dared to pioneer new techniques and therapies which went far beyond what most people thought possible with Alternative medicine. The outcome of his work has been the achievement of miraculous and unprecedented results. His herbal formulae and 30- Day Cleansing and Detoxification *"Incurables"* Program are used in clinics worldwide to help people heal themselves from degenerative diseases such as Heart Disease, Cancer, Arthritis and A.I.D.S. The positive results have caused reverberations in both the natural and medical communities.

A PASSIONATE ELECTRIFYING TEACHER

Dr. Schulze assisted and taught for the late Dr. John Christopher. After Dr. Christopher's death, Dr. Schulze continued to teach at his school for over 12 years. He has served as the Director of The College of Herbology and Natural Healing in the United Kingdom for 11 years and is also Co-Director of The Osho School for Naturopathic Medicine in England, France and Spain. Dr. Schulze has taught and lectured at numerous universities including Cambridge and Oxford Universities in England, Trinity Medical College in Ireland, Omega Institute in New York, Cortijo Romero in Spain and other natural therapy and herbal institutes worldwide. He has been the guest speaker at numerous churches and also on numerous radio and television shows. He is loved for his intensity, passion, dedication to students, sense of humor, creativity, and his exciting, enthusiastic and evangelistic teaching style. He is mostly recognized for his unequaled understanding of natural healing. He continues to teach throughout the United States, Canada, Europe and Asia.

THE AMERICAN BOTANICAL PHARMACY

After 15 years of manufacturing his own herbal formulations in his clinic, Dr. Schulze opened the American Botanical Pharmacy in 1994 which manufactures and sells his industrial-strength, pharmaceutical grade botanical extracts.

Dr. Schulze continues his healing mission today through his daily work to reveal the truth about the unlimited healing power of our being. He is also a leader in exposing fraud in medical, pharmaceutical and even herbal industries. He records numerous audio and video tapes, writes many books and booklets and publishes his free GET WELL Newsletter, all through Natural Healing Publications.